THE SPICE OF VEGETARIAN COOKING

By the same author
Fast Vegetarian Feasts
Gourmet Vegetarian Feasts
The Vegetarian Feast

THE SPICE OF VEGETARIAN COOKING

Ethnic recipes from India, China, Mexico, Southeast Asia, the Middle East, and Europe.

MARTHA ROSE SHULMAN

Illustrated by Elaine Hill

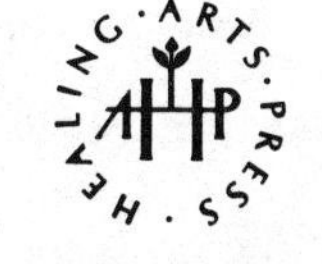

Healing Arts Press
Rochester, Vermont

Healing Arts Press
One Park Street
Rochester, Vermont 05767

Note to the reader: This book is intended as an informational guide. The remedies, approaches, and techniques described herein are meant to supplement, and not to be a substitute for, professional medical care or treatment. They should not be used to treat a serious ailment without prior consultation with a qualified healthcare professional.

LIBRARY OF CONGRESS CATALOGING-IN-PUBLICATION DATA

Shulman, Martha Rose.
[Spicy vegetarian feasts]
The spice of vegetarian cooking : ethnic recipes from India, China, Mexico, Southeast Asia, the Middle East, and Europe / Martha Rose Shulman.
p. cm.
Reprint. Originally published: Spicy vegetarian feasts. Wellingborough; New York : Thorsons, 1986.
Includes bibliographical references and index.
ISBN 0-89281-399-7
1. Cookery (Herbs). 2. Spices. 3. Vegetarian cookery. I. Title.
[TX819.H4S59 1990]
641.6'383—dc20 90–24313
CIP

Printed and bound in the United States

10 9 8 7 6 5 4 3

Healing Arts Press is a division of Inner Traditions International

Distributed to the book trade in Canada by Publishers Group West (PGW), Montreal West, Quebec

Distributed to the health food trade in Canada by Alive Books, Toronto and Vancouver

In memory of my mother, Carol Rees Shulman

CONTENTS

ACKNOWLEDGMENTS

While researching this book, I had the pleasure of reading Julie Sahni's marvelous *Classic Indian Cooking* (William Morrow & Co., New York, 1980); and I feel forever indebted to Mrs. Sahni, not only a wonderful cook but a captivating writer, for helping me understand the rich and varied cuisine of that huge country. In so doing she has also taught me much about the country itself (and given me a good dose of the travel bug to go there).

I am equally grateful to Madhur Jaffrey, whose seemingly endless collections *Eastern Vegetarian Cooking* (Jonathan Cape, London, 1983) and *World of the East Vegetarian Cooking* (Alfred A. Knopf, New York, 1981) increased my desire to visit not only India but also every other Asian country. Both of these cooks, as well as Elizabeth David, have been an inspiration.

I am *most* grateful to my close friend and efficient assistant, Laurie Dill, who helped me with much of the editorial work and carefully tested almost all of the recipes in this book. Laurie is a great cook in her own right, and her suggestions for improvements on many of the recipes have been invaluable.

FOREWORD

It is very frustrating to write a short book on spice cookery as I have done here. Once I began my research I wanted to delve deeply into every cuisine, for spices are in use all over the world—they are the ingredients that give many cuisines their special characters. It is often through the use of spices that cooks have given their personal stamp to their recipes, and I would have liked to experiment to the hilt with my own, to research and cook with those of others to a greater extent, to embark upon the same kind of voyage that brought fifteenth- and sixteenth-century explorers to new continents in search of these very seasonings.

Space and time have not allowed me to do this. What I hope to provide you with here is a small collection of recipes that will familiarize you with spices you may never have used before and that will broaden your repertoire if you are acquainted with these fragrant, magic ingredients. It is an attempt to make the world of cookery a little smaller and to bring a little of India, China, Mexico, Southeast Asia, and the Middle East, as well as Europe and the United States, together in your kitchen.

INTRODUCTION

"... Who knows which palaces, now crumbling to their ruin on the Grand Canal, were indirectly subsidized by the spice-hungry English."

—Elizabeth David
Spices, Salt and Aromatics in the English Kitchen

Until fairly recently the spice cabinet I have in my kitchen today would have made me a rich woman. For 5,000 years, through the end of the Renaissance, spices played the same role in the world economy that petroleum plays today. Spices came to Europe over difficult land routes or treacherous sea routes from India. If I had lived in the thirteenth century, I could have paid my rent, my taxes, and even my dowry in peppercorns; a pound of ginger would have bought me a sheep; two pounds of mace was worth a cow; and a pound of nutmeg was worth seven fat oxen. It was the spice trade that prompted the great sea explorations of the late fifteenth and sixteenth centuries. Were it not for the demand for these seasonings, Vasco da Gama might have stayed at home, or at least continued to take the long route from Portugal to India. Christopher Columbus might never have discovered America, and Europe would not have known the pleasures of the spices, flavorings, and foods indigenous to the New World (allspice, chili peppers, vanilla, chocolate, potatoes, and tomatoes, to name a few) until much later.

The word "spice" has the same root as the word "species," meaning "classes of object." Spices are the aromatic parts—buds, bark, berries, fruit, seeds, roots, or (in the case of saffron) flower stigmas—of certain plants, most of which are indigenous to hot or tropical countries. To Westerners, spices have always seemed exotic because they come, for the most part, from so far away.

The seeds of several herb plants, such as coriander, anise, and fennel, are considered spices; this is where herbs and spices overlap. In this collection you will find some of these seeds (cumin, caraway, and fennel, for example), which I also listed in my *Herbs and Honey Cookery*. I have seen these spices, as well as the capsicum peppers, listed in herbals, but they are considered by most to be spices. There seems to be a great deal of confusion as to the difference between herbs and spices. According to some, culinary herbs are one group of spices. I would define herbs as the leaves of annual and perennial plants which can be used fresh or dried to season dishes, as opposed to spices, which are usually, with the exception of ginger root, used in their dried state.

In any case, spices have been around for thousands of years. Ginger is mentioned in Chinese texts as far back as the fifth century B.C., and spices are well documented in ancient Hindu texts that date from Vedic times (third to first centuries B.C.). Egyptians imported cinnamon and cassia, essential elements in the embalming process, from the East during the Pyramid Age. In ancient times they were the basic ingredients of incense, embalming preservatives, ointments, cosmetics, perfumes, antidotes against poisons, and medicines. The Greeks imported pepper, cassia, cinnamon, ginger, anise, caraway, poppy seeds, fennel, coriander, mint, and garlic from the Far East through Alexandria, the most important trading center between the Mediterranean Sea and the Indian Ocean. Hippocrates mentioned most of these in his medical treatises; over 400 of his preparations are still in use today.

It was not until the first century B.C. in Rome that spices began to be used to a greater extent in cooking. During the time of Pliny (who complained in his writings of the cost of pepper; he apparently didn't feel it was worth it) the use of spices as condiments and seasonings increased greatly, and consumption skyrocketed. Rome developed a very active spice trade with southern Arabia, Somaliland, and India. There was a constant drain of gold to the East for these gastronomic treasures, which were indeed luxury items by the time they reached Rome. Once there, their prices had inflated by 100 times. This was due to shipwrecks, storms, robberies, and—perhaps most important—the greed of the Arab middlemen, who imposed tremendous tariffs and tolls on the spice importers, who were obliged to pass through Arabia on their journey back to Rome. The Arabs controlled the trade routes until the latter half of the first century A.D. They protected their interests by shrouding the origins of the spices in great mystery, maintaining that spices like cinnamon and cassia came from swampy African habitats guarded by huge, ferocious, winged, batlike creatures. Stories like these discouraged importers from attempting to make contact themselves with the real places of origin: China, India, and Asia. But during the latter half of the first century A.D., the Greek merchant Hippalus figured out the seasonal nature of the monsoons in the Indian Ocean, which facilitated sea travel from

Roman Egypt to India. From then on sailors knew that if they made the voyage from Egypt to India between April and October and the return trip between October and April, they could accomplish the round trip in one year instead of two. It was no longer advantageous to go overland. This broke the Arab monopoly, and spices came pouring into the Empire. The Romans became even more extravagant in their use of the condiments; the nobles even slept on saffron-filled pillows because this was believed to be an antidote to the terrible hangovers brought on by their sweet, heavily spiced wines.

Roman imperialism brought spices to the hands of the Goths, Vandals, and Huns. Apparently the barbarians knew their value; for when the Gothic king Alaric made a deal with the Romans in 408 A.D. not to sack the city of Rome, along with his demands for gold, silver, silk tunics, and valuable skins, he demanded 3,000 pounds of peppercorns.

During the Dark Ages there was very little trading between Europe and the East because the Arabs had occupied Alexandria in 641, and the trade routes were no longer safe for European Christians. Mohammed himself had been an experienced spice merchant, having worked as a youth with a Meccan tradesman who dealt in spices with Syria and South Arabia. But the Crusades reopened trade with the East in the eleventh, twelfth, and thirteenth centuries. This is when Venice, whose importance as a port and commercial center was unparalleled, began to rise to the heights it would reach during the early Renaissance.

During the Middle Ages spices were used to mask the odors of decaying food and the putrefying fumes that hung over European towns. There was little variation in the diets of medieval Europeans. They ate no fruits or vegetables to speak of; they ate mainly meat, fowl, and hard, dry bread. The meat, more often than not, was not fresh. Even today the demand for spices is highest in those countries where there is no refrigeration.

But during the Renaissance the standard of living in Europe improved, cooking and eating habits changed, and spices, which had been considered luxuries up until this time, became necessities. Perhaps the European imagination was captured by Marco Polo, who stimulated the Age of Exploration with his descriptions of Kublai Khan's court; his reports recounted numerous delectable, spicy repasts. Europeans became hungrier and hungrier for these exotic ingredients; and merchants and governments, greedier. Spices played the major role in the commercial prosperity of this age.

By the middle of the fifteenth century, land routes to the East had become unsafe again because of the fall of Constantinople to the Turks. The Muslims were imposing extremely high tariffs on spices, and it became imperative for Europeans to open up new sea routes to the East if they wanted an economic future. The kings of Portugal and Spain encouraged sea exploration, and so began the Age of Exploration. At this time Christopher Columbus, convinced he could reach India by sailing west, discovered America; and Vasco da Gama sailed from Portugal around the Cape of Good Hope and on to India. The message he brought home from the king of India stated, "... My country is rich in cinnamon, cloves, ginger, pepper, and precious stones. That which I ask in exchange is gold, silver, corals, and scarlet cloth." A fleet was fitted out immediately and was sent off. So ended the Venetian monopoly on spices, and thus began the European monopoly. Cinnamon, cloves, and peppercorns would never again finance a doge's palace.

For the next 200 years the price of spices would serve as a barometer for the world economy, and the European demand would stimulate more exploration and colonization. Expeditions such as Magellan's circumnavigation of the globe from 1519 to 1522 and Cortes' conquest of Mexico in 1519 usually returned with only a handful of the men they had set out with, but always with the hulls of whatever ships remained packed with tons of cloves, nutmegs, mace, and cinnamon as well as gold and silver.

It seems that almost all of the European countries profited from the spice trade (but not without inflicting savagely cruel, slavelike conditions on the natives of the countries they colonized). The English founded the East India Company in 1600. The Dutch, who grew rich by providing ships and crews and eventually began to expand their own trade to the Far East, founded the United Dutch East India Company in 1602 and eventually drove the Portuguese out of the Spice Islands. By the end of the seventeenth century the Dutch controlled the spice trade, only to be defeated by the British a century later.

By the end of the eighteenth century the United States had entered the market, especially in the West Indies, but also in Sumatra. From 1800 to 1811 Salem, Massachusetts, monopolized the Sumatra pepper trade, bringing in from 500 to as much as 1,200 tons a year.

But by the middle of the seventeenth century spices were no longer luxury items as they were so much easier to obtain, nor were they necessary for masking the rancid flavors of foods as now there was much more variety. In eighteenth-century England the use of spices became a kind of fad, which Restoration playwrights did not hesitate to mock. We can still find pocket nutmeg graters and Georgian cinnamon casters dating from this time. People carried spices to season the heavily spiced drinks, which were then the rage.

Modern times have seen a decrease in the use of spices in the West as food has become industrialized and synthetic spice essences and flavorings have begun to be manufactured. This is a pity, as nothing can really imitate their distinctive flavors. But recently, perhaps because of the influx of Asian and Latin American populations into Europe and North America, there has been a growing interest in exotic cuisines like Indian, Chinese, Mexican, Vietnamese, Thai, and North African—the cuisines that make the most of spices. We in the West have always been comfortable with the sweet dessert spices like cinnamon, nutmeg, and cloves; but, on the whole, we are not altogether at home with spices like cardamom, turmeric, and cumin. Now that the world has become so small and spices of all kinds are quite easy to come by, they needn't remain a mystery.

Cooking with Spices

The way to become comfortable with spices is to work with them, to become familiar with each one, and to learn the way they act upon the foods they are seasoning as well as how they interact with one another. Each spice has unique and specific properties. Some are aromatics, some add heat to a dish, and some lend coloring. Others are souring agents, and still others act as thickeners. Some spices have more than one property; saffron, for example, is used to color dishes, and, at the same time, it lends a marvelous sweet aroma. Only a handful of spices are "hot," though when we use the word "spicy," hot is what we usually mean. Spices vary in fragrance, sweetness, aroma, and heat. Sometimes a particular spice is intended to dominate a dish; at other times several are meant to blend together in a dish and not overwhelm. Despite the fact that "spicy" has strong connotations to most people, some of the most successfully spiced dishes are very subtle. Spices are usually added to dishes in relatively small amounts.

Most spices must be cooked before they will release their fragrance. They release more of their aroma when slightly crushed.

In addition to culinary properties, spices, like herbs, have healing and medicinal properties. In Indian cuisine these properties have influenced their use in certain kinds of dishes. Asafetida and ginger root counteract flatulence and colic so they are often added to leguminous preparations. Fennel, cardamom, and cloves stimulate the digestive system, curb nausea, and provide relief from heartburn and indigestion so they are chewed after Indian meals. Cloves act as an antiseptic and are often used in pickles. Fenugreek water is used as a tonic for gastritis and other stomach disorders; the soaked seeds are a very effective digestive aid, and, for this reason, they are often added to Indian dahls and starchy vegetable dishes.

Spices also have an effect on body temperature. "Warm spices" generate internal body heat and are recommended for cold weather. We find the warm spices—cardamom, cinnamon, powdered ginger, mace, nutmeg, and hot red pepper—in the cuisines of the mountainous regions of Northern India. "Cool spices" take away body heat. All the spices which are not "warm" range from "very cool" to "moderately warm." The after-dinner spices are all "cool."

One reason we find spicy dishes in hot, tropical countries is that in addition to the fact that these are the regions in which the spices grow, spices induce perspiration, which has a cooling effect. That's one reason why people in India drink hot tea laced with spices even in very hot weather.

The reason people sometimes have digestive problems after eating spiced food is that most spices are not easily digestible in the raw form. For this reason they should either be cooked in oil or simmered with food, or if added to an uncooked dish, they should be dry-roasted first (although I often add very small amounts of uncooked spices like cumin, curry powder, and chili powder to uncooked foods like guacamole and salad dressings).

When a recipe calls for several spices, you should measure them out and have them ready by the stove before beginning to cook.

Buying, Storing, and Grinding

Spices, like coffee, are infinitely more aromatic and complex if bought whole and freshly ground when you use them. Whole, they will remain fresh for up to one year if properly stored in sealed jars in a cool, dry, dark place. Asafetida, mustard seeds, and fenugreek will stay fresh for up to three years.

Once spices are ground, their aromatic oils begin to evaporate. It takes only minutes to grind your own. I keep an extra coffee mill for spices. *Never* use your only coffee mill for spices. I learned this the first time I used my coffee mill to grind cinnamon sticks and cloves. From then on my coffee always tasted as if it were laced with spices because the blades and plastic cover retained some of the oils and resins of the spices (apparently these are more powerful than those in the coffee beans), and I was quickly obliged to buy myself another mill for coffee.

A recipe will often call for a small amount of a crushed spice or seeds. This is easily done with a mortar and pestle. Ceramic mortars like the Japanese suribachi and marble or brass mortars are the most efficient for this. You can also use a kitchen mallet or rolling pin. First place the spice in a plastic bag, and then pound on a flat surface.

For peppercorns my favorite mill is the kind you can adjust so that the pepper can be coarse or fine depending on the recipe. There are also handy mills on the market that have a container on the bottom for quick measuring.

Some beautiful nutmeg graters are now available that are engineered like a peppermill but with a small blade on the bottom that shaves the nutmeg and grates them down to the last flake. Standard nutmeg graters do the job too, of course, but with more damage to your fingers or knuckles when you get down to the end of the nutmeg. Look for the kind with a container for storing the nutmeg.

The French company SEB is now distributing its Minichop abroad. This has a detachable blade which makes for easy cleaning, but it doesn't powder as finely as a coffee mill does, and, like the electric coffee mill, the plastic container and blades will retain the resin and aroma of the spices—so don't plan on using your Minichop for garlic and herbs as well as spices.

There are also attractive hand grinders on the market. They look like small grain mills which latch onto the edge of a table and are handy for grinding large amounts of spices.

Food processors and blenders don't grind spices finely enough. My choice is the electric coffee mill, which is inexpensive and efficient.

Roasting Spices

Often recipes, especially for several Indian dishes, call for roasted, ground spices. These are roasted in a dry, heavy frying pan or griddle until they turn dark brown. To roast spices, heat an Indian griddle ("kadhai") or a dry, heavy frying pan, preferably cast iron, for two minutes over medium heat. Add the spices and roast over medium heat, stirring constantly and shaking the pan so they don't burn. For the first minute or two nothing will happen, then suddenly the spices will begin to jump around, brown, and smoke. Watch very carefully and stir constantly. Lower the heat a little if they seem to be browning too fast. When they are dark brown, they are done. Transfer immediately to a cool, dry bowl and allow to cool. Grind, if instructed, to a fine powder in an electric or hand mill. The roasting time will depend on the size of the pan and the amount of spice as well as the kind of spice. On a standard Indian griddle 4 tablespoons of coriander seeds take 6 minutes, 4 tablespoons of cumin seeds take 8 minutes, and 1½ cups of garam masala, 10 minutes.

Frying Spices

In many Indian recipes spices are fried in hot oil or fat to remove their raw taste and release their flavor into the oil before the other ingredients are added. The oil must be hot enough to allow the spices to brown quickly but not so hot that they'll burn. Because I use less fat in my cooking than traditional Indian cooks, I fry the spices at a lower temperature for slightly longer to avoid burning. The results are the same; the perfume of the spices penetrates the other foods in the dish.

Whole spices should always be added to a dish before ground spices, and the heat should be a little lower for ground spices. Mustard seeds and fenugreek cook more slowly than other spices in their whole state. When mustard seeds are fried they pop like popcorn, which releases their flavor. Unpopped they are chewy and bitter. When frying mustard seeds in oil, have a lid handy to protect yourself from sputtering seeds and oil.

Freezing Spiced Food

When food is frozen, the ice crystals rupture cell walls and flavor constituents are released. For this reason, spicy foods will be spicier if frozen and thawed. This is something to consider when you are making piquant foods for the freezer. Be cautious with your peppery ingredients; you can always add more after you've tested the thawed dish.

A GLOSSARY OF SPICES

Some of the spices I have listed here also appear in my *Herb and Honey Cookery* (Thorsons, 1984). As I explained earlier in this section, this is because there seems to be some confusion as to whether the seeds of certain herb plants, like cumin and caraway, fall under the category of herbs or spices; and I have seen these, as well as the capsicum peppers, listed in herbals. But having read numerous definitions of spices since beginning this book, I now concede that those ingredients which I also listed in my herb book are indeed spices.

ALLSPICE

Whole allspice (or pimento) berries are the fruits of the *Pimenta dioica* tree, native to the West Indies and Latin America. The round berries, slightly larger than peppercorns, are picked green and are dried in the sun, whereupon they take on their rusty-brown color. As with all spices, it is best to purchase allspice berries whole and grind them as you use them.

Outside the United States allspice is known as **pimento** because the Spaniards, thinking the berries resembled peppercorns in flavor, named the spice pimiento when they discovered it in the West Indies. It is the only major spice grown on a commercial basis exclusively in the Western Hemisphere. Most of it (and the best) is grown in Jamaica, although it is also grown in Guatemala, Brazil, Mexico, Honduras, and the Leeward Islands.

The name allspice derives from the flavor of this sweet, fragrant spice, which is reminiscent of several of the sweet spices, most notably cinnamon and cloves, with a hint of nutmeg and pepper.

The spice is used all over the world to sweeten and spice baked goods, as a pickling spice, and in many Middle Eastern dishes. It can surprise the palate in the most pleasing way when it occurs in a Moroccan carrot, beet, or orange salad.

ANAHEIM CHILI

These are also known as the California chili, the chile verde, the long green chili, and Big Jim (all different chilies but close enough to be interchanged in recipes). They are long, narrow, and slightly twisted with colors ranging from light to dark green and sometimes ripened to yellow, orange, and red. The flavor is peppery and fresh, ranging from mild to hot. They are found in most American markets and are good stuffed or minced to add spice to various dishes.

ANISE SEEDS

Anise seeds are native to Asia Minor, the Greek Islands, and Egypt and were used by the ancient Egyptians, Greeks, and Romans to sweeten and flavor food and beverages. They have a sweet, licorice flavor and are used as a flavoring for candy, breads, and other baked goods. They are also the flavoring agent for the various licorice-flavored liqueurs and cordials popular all over the Mediterranean. Pastis, anisette, ouzo, and arak are all flavored with anise as well as with fennel and star anise. The ground seeds are also often an ingredient in Indian curries, particularly vegetarian and fish dishes from Bengal. The seeds, slightly roasted, are chewed after Indian meals to aid digestion.

ASAFETIDA

This strange ingredient is used in very small amounts in Indian cooking. It is a combination of various dried gum resins of Indian and Iranian plants and can be bought in lump and powdered form in Indian markets. Buy the lump form if possible because asafetida does not release its rather unpleasant odor (not unlike bad garlic or onions) unless it is powdered.

A lump of asafetida about the size of a pea will undergo a mysterious change when heated in oil; the aroma and flavor mellow and resemble mild onions. It is used in the cuisine of the strictest Hindu sects, who believe that onions and garlic are too strong and that the two should never be used together.

CAPSICUM PEPPERS

This family of peppers, indigenous to the New World, includes cayenne, the hot peppers used in Asian cuisines, those used in Mexican cooking, and the different grades of Hungarian paprika. It is a very diverse family because the peppers breed prodigiously and crossbreed easily (there are over 200 capsicum peppers in existence, of which 100 can be found in Mexico alone); so it can be very confusing, especially since some of the names change when the peppers are used in their dried state.

The heat of the various capsicum peppers varies from one to the other. It seems that the smaller peppers are the most fiery. Some of those used in Indonesian and Asian cuisines outstrip the Mexican peppers by a long shot; I'm always flabbergasted by how much heat can be contained in one speck of a little pepper. There is also great variation in our tolerance for hot peppers. This seems to be genetic; some people can gobble down whole jalapeños without blinking an eye, whereas others take one bite and are in agony—their noses run, their eyes water, and their palate is finished for the evening. Research has recently shown that hot peppers trigger the release of endorphins, which may explain why some people seem to get so high from them. As for antidotes for the heat, water is of no use whatsoever. I've had the best luck eating a piece of bread, which seems to absorb some of the heat.

The following are those most commonly used in Mexican, European, and Asian cuisines (there are many more peppers that you would come across in markets in Mexico and Asian countries, but these are the ones you can find outside these countries).

CARAWAY SEEDS

These seeds have a distinctive flavor I always associate with Jewish rye bread. People either like the flavor or hate it so it's best not to serve dishes heavily seasoned with the seeds to people whose tastes are not familiar to you. They are a common ingredient in German and Austrian cuisines. I love the seeds in breads, potato or grain soups, and some salads.

CARDAMOM SEEDS

These are small, black, fragrant seeds which come in black, green, or white pods (white pods are actually green pods which have been bleached). Black cardamom, which is more fragrant than green cardamom, is only available in specialty stores and Indian markets. Green cardamom can always be substituted for black. Cardamom has a distinctive earthy-perfume flavor and aroma. One of the key ingredients in Mughal garam masala, it is commonly used in Indian dishes as well as in spice breads and cakes. The whole pods are often added to pilafs and vegetable dishes; they give off their marvelous aroma as the dishes cook. They are not meant to be eaten in this whole state, but no harm will be done if they are.

CAROM

Carom is the seed of the lovage plant and is used in Indian dishes. The seeds look like celery seeds and have a sharp, hot taste and thyme-like aroma. It is sold in Indian grocery stores and is used as a flavoring in Indian vegetable dishes, breads, and savory pastries.

CAYENNE

In Mexico and India this pepper is used fresh. It is mid-green and is about 3 inches long and ¾ inch wide. For the most part, though, it is ripened to red and is usually used in its dried state, either whole, crushed, or ground. It is extremely hot—a little goes a long way. Just a few grains will add heat to any dish. You will find it in most of the spicy Indian recipes, and it is a must in Cajun cuisine.

CHILE CASCABEL

A small, round, dried Mexican chili with a brownish-red, smooth skin. It sounds like a rattle when you shake it. It is less "picante" than the guajillo and has a nice, nutty flavor when toasted and ground for sauces.

CHILE GUAJILLO

A long, pointed, slender, dried Mexican chili averaging 4½ inches long and 1¼ inches wide. It is extremely "picante."

CHILE JALAPEÑO

This is the other small, green chili most often used in its fresh or pickled state in Mexican dishes. Jalapeños are mid- to dark-green with a smooth surface and a more rounded tip than the serrano. They are about 2 ½ inches long on the average and about ¾ inch wide at the widest part, a fatter chili than the serrano. They are quite hot but not quite as vibrantly "picante" as the serrano. I use them interchangeably for salsas and other Mexican preparations.

Jalapeños can be stored in the same way as serranos. They are fairly easy to find canned in *escabeche* and are widely used in this form as a condiment with Mexican food. They are also quite good stuffed (see recipe, page 149). Fresh or canned, jalapeños are a necessary garnish for *nachos* (see page 144).

When jalapeños are ripened and smoked, they become *chiles chipotles*. These can be found in escabeche or in a red *adobo* sauce (they are the most popular in this pickled state) or dried—available in stores that sell Mexican ingredients. They have a distinctive piquant, smoky flavor.

Jalapeños can be used in all recipes calling for hot, green chili peppers.

CHILE MULATO

Another dried Mexican chili roughly the same shape as the *ancho* but with a tougher, slightly less wrinkled skin. It is brownish black and often difficult to distinguish from the *ancho*. The flavor is a bit sweeter than that of the *ancho*.

CHILE PASILLA

This is the dried form of the *chile chilaca,* a long, slim, very dark green chili averaging 6 inches in length and 1 inch wide. It is very hot and has a rich, dusky flavor. It is used in combination with the chile ancho in sauces like mole (page 150). Because of its dark, almost black color, the chili pasilla is sometimes referred to as the *chile negro.*

CHILE POBLANO

These are large, undulating, triangular-shaped peppers with a dark green (sometimes almost black), shiny skin. Their size averages about 3 inches wide at the top and 5 inches long, tapering down to a point. Although poblanos can be quite "picante," on the average they are relatively mild, and their flavor is very rich and aromatic. They are usually roasted and peeled before using (this enhances their flavor even more) and are used for the stuffed chilies ("chiles rellenos") in Mexican and Southwestern cuisines. Roasted and cut into strips, they become "rajas," which are used in many vegetable dishes and casseroles. Once roasted and peeled, they can be frozen in plastic bags and used as needed.

When dried, the chile poblano becomes the *chile ancho.* These have a deep reddish-brown color and a wrinkled skin. The basis for many of the red chili sauces in Mexican and Southwestern cooking (see mole sauce, page 150), they are probably the most widely used chili in Mexico.

CHILE SECO

Another dried chili from the Yucatan and Campeche regions of Mexico. These taste a little like hot paprika, which can be substituted for the peppers. They are small and bright red.

CHILE SERRANO

These are small, narrow, dark green chilies (sometimes they ripen to red) about 1½ inches long on the average and a little less than ½ inch wide. They are used in many Mexican recipes (see the salsas on page 138, for instance) and are very hot with a fresh, vibrant flavor. They will keep for several weeks if kept dry and stored at the bottom of the refrigerator. Separate out any that are soft or turning bad, and wrap the rest in a paper towel. Do not keep in a plastic bag as they will release moisture and rot sooner. The peppers may wrinkle, but they will still be good.

Chilies serranos can also be frozen. First toast them in a dry frying pan or on a griddle until the skin blisters and turns brown and they are soft, or boil them in water for 10 minutes and then drain. Freeze in plastic bags, and use as needed.

Ripened, dried serranos are sold as *serranos secos* or *chile japones*. They are also sold canned in a pickling medium called *escabeche*.

Serranos can be used in all recipes calling for small, hot, green chilies.

CHINESE FIVE SPICE

This is a Chinese mixture of equal parts ground anise pepper (a close relative of anise with a more pungent flavor), star anise, cassia (a close relative of cinnamon, also with a more pungent flavor), cloves, and fennel seed. The mixture has a sweet, subtle flavor and is an ingredient in many Oriental dishes. It can be found in Chinese and Vietnamese groceries, or you can make it yourself.

CHINESE HOT PEPPER OIL

Oil seasoned with Chinese hot peppers, extremely hot, and found in Chinese groceries.

Dried peppers will keep indefinitely if they have been dried under good conditions and are stored in a cool, dry place. Check every few months and remove any that may be deteriorating. I store mine in large, tightly sealed jars in the pantry.

CHINESE HOT PEPPERS

These are used in hot Szechuan and Hunan dishes and can be pretty fiery. Sometimes you can find them in flake form or ground form in Chinese groceries. In authentic regional Chinese cooking, specific peppers from each region are used, but these are not always easy to find. If you can't find Chinese peppers, substitute cayenne. Mexican peppers would be too sweet.

CINNAMON AND CASSIA

These are both sold interchangeably as cinnamon, although they are derived from different trees. They have almost identical sweet, pungent flavors, cassia being slightly more pungent, and are used in the West to flavor sweets and baked foods, syrups, hot mulled ciders, wines, and punches. In Indian cooking cinnamon is an important ingredient in pilafs and is one of the ingredients in Mughal garam masala (page 26). I use it to heighten the flavors of an Italian tomato sauce: a tiny pinch of cinnamon added just at the end brings out the sweetness of the tomatoes and the aroma of the garlic and other herbs. It's a trick that surprises many people, but it always works.

Cinnamon and cassia are the barks of the cinnamon and cassia trees. The spices are at their best when freshly ground, but for baking it is sometimes difficult to get a fine-enough grind so using powdered cinnamon is preferable. Have both sticks and ground cinnamon on hand, but don't let the powdered cinnamon get too old. Whole sticks of cinnamon are used to flavor Indian pilafs and are removed after cooking.

Cassia is one of the oldest of all spices. It was recorded in China in 2500 B.C. and in Egypt in 1600 B.C. It came into Europe over the spice routes.

CLOVES

Cloves are the dried buds of an evergreen tree native to the Molucca Islands in eastern Indonesia. They have a sweet, strong, pungent flavor and aroma. A little goes a long way. It's best to buy cloves whole and grind them as you need them. In Indian cooking they are used in pilafs and other preparations in their whole and powdered form, and they are an ingredient in Mughal garam masala. They have antiseptic properties, which is one reason why they are an ingredient in pickling. They are commonly used in spiced and mulled wines, ciders and punches, spice breads, and cakes.

CORIANDER SEEDS

These light brown spherical seeds, slightly larger than peppercorns, have a completely different flavor than the fresh leaves of the plant (the leaves are an herb, the seeds, a spice). The flavor is mild and sort of musky-sweet,with a subtle hint of orange peel. They are widely used in Indian cooking, both whole and ground, and are an essential ingredient in garam masala (page 27). In Indian cuisine they are often roasted before being ground (see section on roasting spices, page 7). In their raw, powdered form they can serve as a thickener in Indian sauces and gravies.

In France coriander seeds are an essential ingredient in vegetables cooked *a la Grecque* and in *pain d'epices* (page 46). In English and North American cooking, coriander is an important pickling spice and is found in spice breads and cakes. It also occurs in several Middle Eastern and North African dishes.

CUMIN SEEDS

Cumin seeds in their whole and ground states are an essential ingredient in Mexican, Indian, and North African cuisines. The spice has a very special, unmistakable nutty-earthy aroma. The seeds are light brown in color and resemble caraway seeds in appearance, but their flavor is totally different. Ground, roasted cumin is added to many Indian raitas and appetizers and should be kept on hand (see instructions for roasting and grinding, page 7). I add cumin to several cheese and vegetables dishes (it is especially good with potatoes) and sometimes to breads.

CURRY POWDER

Curry powder is not one spice but is a blend of several spices. The name derives from the Indian word "kari," which can mean either the sweet aromatic leaves of the kari plant (used in southern and southwestern Indian regional cooking) or a south Indian technique of preparing stir-fried vegetables, which involves a spice blend called "kari podi" (curry powder). The classic kari podi blend includes roasted ground turmeric, red pepper, coriander, black pepper, cumin, fenugreek, kari leaves, mustard seeds, and sometimes cinnamon and cloves. The earliest British merchants who colonized

India probably took this powder back to England with them so they could mimic the flavors and aromas they had grown fond of in India. Without much knowledge or understanding of authentic Indian cuisine, they would add this powder to meat and vegetable dishes, which eventually became known as curries. As English influence spread into the north and east of India, new ingredients found their way into curry powder, while at the same time the word "curry" became very popular within the English-speaking Indian middle class. Eventually, simple Indian dishes with spices gravies, known as "salans," became known as curries even though these dishes bear no resemblance to the dishes we in the West know by that name.

In true Indian cuisine the balance of fresh spices is so important that curry powder would never work, especially since curry powders vary in heat and pungency and often contain ingredients never used in certain regional dishes. Indians do use premixed blends—garam masala and Mughal garam masala—but these are used only as a base for spicing a dish (see pages 26–27).

The European curry powders can, however, lend a very pleasant flavor to a dish, and I use this seasoning frequently. Care must be taken, though, when purchasing curry powders as some are much hotter and fresher than others. Bad curry powders taste bitter, like little more than turmeric. This is one spice worth looking for in the best imported spice shops.

The ingredients most often used in curry powders are the following: black pepper, dried red chilies, cloves, cinnamon, cardamom, coriander seeds, cumin seeds, curry leaves, fenugreek seeds, dried ginger (sometimes), mace or nutmeg (sometimes), mustard seeds, and turmeric.

FENNEL SEEDS

These seeds of the fennel herb plant have a licorice flavor like anise and can be used interchangeably. They are not quite so strong as anise. Fennel has been cultivated in India since Vedic times and is also native to southern

Europe; it was popular among the Romans, who spread it to other parts of the continent.

FENUGREEK SEEDS

The seeds of fenugreek, an annual herb which is a member of the bean family, are native to Asia Minor and India. Fenugreek is an important ingredient in Indian cooking. The small, hard, vaguely triangular seeds have a very strong aroma and bitter taste. Recipes call for a very few, and they impart a distinctive curry flavor. They are known to be a digestive and for this reason are often cooked with legumes.

GINGER

In its fresh state ginger root is one of my favorite spices. It is pungent and aromatic without being overwhelmingly piquant and finds its place in all kinds of dishes—soups, vegetables, grains, tofu dishes, salads, and desserts. Entire cook books have been devoted to this spice. A common ingredient in Indian, Chinese, and Japanese cuisines, it is easy to find in Oriental markets and some supermarkets. Look for smooth unshriveled roots. To prepare fresh ginger, peel and thinly slice, then chop very fine or cut in shreds, depending on the recipe. Fresh, peeled ginger can also be grated or minced in a food processor. To store the root, place it in a jar of sherry in the refrigerator. It will keep indefinitely.

Dried ginger, usually found in its powdered form, has a much different flavor than fresh and is used in different kinds of dishes. In Indian cuisine it is used in Moghul dishes to lend a piquant or sour taste and sweet, woody fragrance. I find the spice rather bitter and try not to substitute it for fresh ginger when that is what a recipe calls for. But dried ginger is a particularly welcome ingredient in many spiced breads and cakes, especially *pain d'epices* (page 46), gingerbread (page 182) and gingersnaps (page 191).

MACE

Mace and nutmeg are both part of the fruit of the nutmeg tree and are native to the Molucca Islands. Mace is the lining of the nutmeg; it is carefully peeled off the shell and dried until it becomes brittle and yellowish brown in color. The dried membranes are sold commercially as mace blades or are ground as mace (as usual, the blades are preferable). Its flavor is similar to that of nutmeg but stronger, and the two should not be used interchangeably. Mace is an ingredient in several Indian and Kashmiri dishes and is a spice in several European and American cakes and sweets.

MANGO POWDER

This is derived from dried, unripened mangos which are ground to a buff-colored powder. The powder has a pungent aroma and is used to impart a sour taste to certain Indian dishes.

MUSTARD SEEDS

Two kinds of mustard seeds are commonly used. **Black mustard seeds** (also called brown mustard and Indian mustard) look a bit like poppy seeds but are larger. They are indispensable in southern and southwestern Indian cuisines, and they are used as a pickling spice and flavoring for vegetable dishes in north Indian cuisine. The seeds have a pungent aroma and a slightly bitter, slightly sour flavor. They are usually sautéed in hot oil just until they stop sputtering, then are stirred into a dish (such as a dahl) to impart a distinct, yet subtle, tang. They are available in Indian markets.

Yellow or **white mustard seeds** are the seeds ground to make dry mustard powder and all prepared mustards. The pungency of prepared mustards is due to an oil which is released when the seeds are ground or crushed and mixed with water. An enzyme causes the bitter substance in the mustard, glucoside, to react with the water, and the hot flavor emerges. Powdered mustard, therefore, once mixed with cold water, must be allowed to stand for 10 minutes so that the hot flavor can emerge. Boiling water will kill the enzyme, and the resulting mustard will be mild and bitter tasting. Mustard seeds act as a preservative, which is one reason they are widely used in pickling. They have been used as a spice for thousands of years.

NUTMEG

The inner part of the fruit of the nutmeg tree, this spice has a delicious sweet, nutty flavor. It is commonly used in Moghul and Kashmiri cooking and is one of the ingredients in Mughal garam masala (see page 26). In Western cuisines it is one of the sweet spices in baked goods and sweets, but it is also used to season soups, vegetables (especially spinach), cream sauces, and many pasta and cheese dishes. It should always be freshly grated, as it will quickly lose its zesty aroma when powdered. Nutmeg is one of my favorite spices. It gives many of my vegetable fillings for crêpes and pasta a mysterious and wonderful lift, and I often season fruit pastries and desserts with it. It goes especially well with bananas. The spice should be used with discretion, as the flavor can overpower a dish. It is especially useful for those on a salt-free diet.

PAPRIKA

Also known as Hungarian pepper and Spanish pepper, this is the national spice of Hungary. Paprika is the dried powder of a mild, sweet, bright red pepper. It is extremely high in vitamin C and carotene, and it stimulates circulation. It should have a mild, sweet flavor, and you should use it in large quantities, a teaspoon or more at a time. It must be very fresh (if the color has gone from bright red to rust brown, it has deteriorated), or it will be bitter. Store it in the refrigerator in an air-tight container. There are eight grades of Hungarian paprika, ranging from mild and sweet to hot and very rich. Always look for the word "Hungarian" or "Magyar" on the package or, even better, "Kalocsa" or "Szeged," two cities in the heart of the paprika region. **Indian paprika** has a pungent aroma and a sweet taste and is used in many Kashmiri preparations. I use paprika most often in soups, bean dishes, and vegetable dishes.

PEPPERCORNS (BLACK AND WHITE)

Peppercorns, noted over 3,000 years ago in Sanskrit texts for their medicinal and preservative effects, are native to India and found their way from there to China and

Europe. They are by far the most important spice in world trade today, claiming 25 percent of the market; 160 million pounds of peppercorns are sold annually. Although you see black pepper everywhere, you may not be aware of the subtle differences between the different kinds of peppercorns and the different effects of various grinds on the palate. Fine-quality black peppercorns smell and taste richly aromatic and full bodied; poor-quality peppercorns smell musty and one-dimensional. Canned and ground peppercorns are stale and should not even be considered; they have a sharp, metallic taste, and they don't resemble freshly ground pepper at all.

It's amazing how such a commonly used spice can change the face of a dish. A few coarse grinds into a green salad will add an entire dimension as it will to soups and vegetable dishes. In quantity, ground pepper will add fire to a dish. This is the hot ingredient in Chinese hot and sour soup.

There are several varieties of black peppercorns. They are all berries that are picked green, allowed to ferment for several days, and then dried in the sun until shriveled and blackish brown. The core of the berry remains white. *Tellicherry,* from the northern Malabar coast, has a rich aroma and big taste—spicy, but not sharp. *Brazilian,* harvested along the Amazon River, is much like the Tellicherry, with an herbal scent and subtle hotness. *Malabar,* from the southern Malabar coast, is very aromatic and hot, with a slightly minty aftertaste. *Lampong,* from southern Sumatra, is tannic and sharp, with relatively little aroma.

White peppercorns are berries picked when they are fully mature, soaked in water for eight days until soft, and then hulled. The gray inner cores are washed and sun-dried until bleached white. They are hotter than black peppercorns and are less aromatic.

Mignonette pepper is a mix of white and black peppercorns, which brings together the aroma of black and the strength of white pepper. The ratio of black to white is usually four parts black to one part white.

Green peppercorns are picked immature and are marketed in their undried, soft state. They are best bought fresh or freeze-dried or bottled in natural juices (not brine) with no preservatives. They are often mashed to a paste and added to sauces and butters.

Red peppercorns, usually sold freeze-dried or bottled in natural juices, have a marvelous distinctive flavor which is more herbal than spicy. I flavor stuffings, grains, and salads with them.

PEPPERONCINI

This is the hot pepper used in Italian cuisine and pickled and sold as the Italian pickled pepper. The peppers are small, twisted, and pale green.

PICKLING SPICE

The proportions of the different spices vary in pickling spices, but they usually consist of black peppercorns, red chilies, mustard seeds, allspice, cloves, ginger (sometimes), mace, and coriander seeds.

POPPY SEEDS

Most common in or on breads and pastries, these tiny gray-black seeds have a pleasant, nutty flavor when baked. Ground white poppy seeds are used in Indian cooking to thicken gravies. When they are roasted before being ground, the seeds impart to their dishes a pleasant, nutty aroma similar to that of Chinese sesame oil.

SAFFRON

This is the most luxurious and expensive of spices. It is the dried stigmas of the flowers of the saffron plant, a member of the crocus family. It is so costly (it retails over $2,000 a pound!) because it takes about 250,000 dried stigmas, collected from about 75,000 flowers, to make a pound of saffron. It is usually sold by the twentieth of an ounce or by the gram in thread and powdered form. I buy the threads because powdered saffron is often adulterated. In Paris I buy my saffron at the pharmacy, where it is used in some homeopathic preparations.

Saffron's magic lies in the gorgeous yellow hue it imparts to its dishes and its strong, sweet, vaguely sealike aroma. I have sometimes had a hard time convincing strict vegetarians that there is no seafood in my vegetarian paella.

A little of this spice goes a long way, luckily. It takes only ¼ teaspoon to color and flavor a cup of rice. To achieve even coloring and flavoring, powder the saffron threads with your fingers or the back of a spoon in a small bowl and soak in a little hot water or milk for 15 minutes. Add this solution, with the threads, to whatever you are cooking.

STAR ANISE

Star anise, a native of China and important in Chinese cuisine, is the star-shaped fruit of an evergreen tree belonging to the magnolia family. The spice has a licorice flavor that is stronger and slightly more bitter than that of anise. It is an ingredient in Chinese Five Spice and can be found in Oriental markets.

TAMARIND

Although this isn't a spice, but the pulpy pod of a tropical plant, I'm including it in this list because it is often used to impart a sour flavor to Indian dishes. The pulp of the mature tamarind pods is compressed into balls or cakes, which are sold in Indian and Asian grocery stores. Tamarind tastes like very sour prunes. The flavor is extracted by soaking the tamarind in boiling water, then mashing the pulp and straining. This juice is used as a souring agent.

TURMERIC

Turmeric is native to India and belongs to the ginger family. The roots are cleaned, boiled, dried, and ground to a deep ocher-colored powder. It is one of the main ingredients in curry powder. Turmeric imparts a lovely yellow color to dishes and has a woody and, in my opinion, slightly bitter flavor. It is an important sacred spice in Hindu religions.

VANILLA

Not a spice but an aromatic, vanilla lends fragrance to syrups, pastries, and sweet dessert sauces. It is the pod of a climbing orchid native to the rain forests of the New

World. The Aztecs used it as a flavoring for chocolate. We use it to flavor sweet dishes.

Vanilla beans are picked unripe and are cured. They are dark brown with a shiny, flexible, tough skin. To extract their flavor for syrups and sauces, cut them in half lengthwise and simmer the beans, then remove them. Use pure vanilla extract in baked goods.

SPICE BLENDS

In Indian cooking spice blends are called "masalas," which means a blend of several aromatic spices. In Indian homes, masalas are sometimes pastes and are made by grinding herbs and seasonings along with the spices. The masalas are what give regional Indian dishes their distinctive flavors. Authentic garam masalas must be made at home. The following Mughal garam masala and garam masala are Julie Sahni's blend, from her *Classic Indian Cooking* (William Morrow & Co., 1980).

MUGHAL GARAM MASALA

This is essential to most North Indian preparations. It is usually added to a dish at the end, just before serving, to enhance the flavors of other ingredients. In some recipes, however, it is added at the beginning. This blend is subtle and mellow, with a cardamom flavor. In India it is used in cream-, milk-, yogurt-, and fruit-sauce-based dishes.

Makes 12 tablespoons or ¾ cup

½ cup (about 60) black, or ⅓ cup (about 20) green or white cardamom pods
2 cinnamon sticks, 3 inches long
1 tablespoon whole cloves
1 tablespoon black peppercorns
1½ teaspoons grated nutmeg (optional)

Remove the seeds from the cardamom pods. Crush the cinnamon stick with a kitchen mallet or rolling pin and combine with the other spices, except the nutmeg, and grind to a fine powder. Mix in the grated nutmeg, if desired. Store in an airtight container in a cool place.

Garam Masala

This is a more pungent, spicy version of the masala, containing large quantities of coriander and cumin. It is used in North Indian cooking. If you wish to make this hotter, increase the amount of peppercorns.

Makes 12 tablespoons or ¾ cup

- *1½ tablespoons (about 10) black or 1 tablespoon green cardamom pods*
- *3 cinnamon sticks, 3 inches long*
- *1½ teaspoons whole cloves*
- *2 tablespoons black peppercorns*
- *4 tablespoons cumin seeds*
- *4 tablespoons coriander seeds*

Remove the seeds from the cardamom pods. Crush the cinnamon with a kitchen mallet or rolling pin and combine with the other spices. Roast them in a dry frying pan or griddle (see roasting instructions, page 7), and grind to a fine powder. Store in an air-tight container in a cool place.

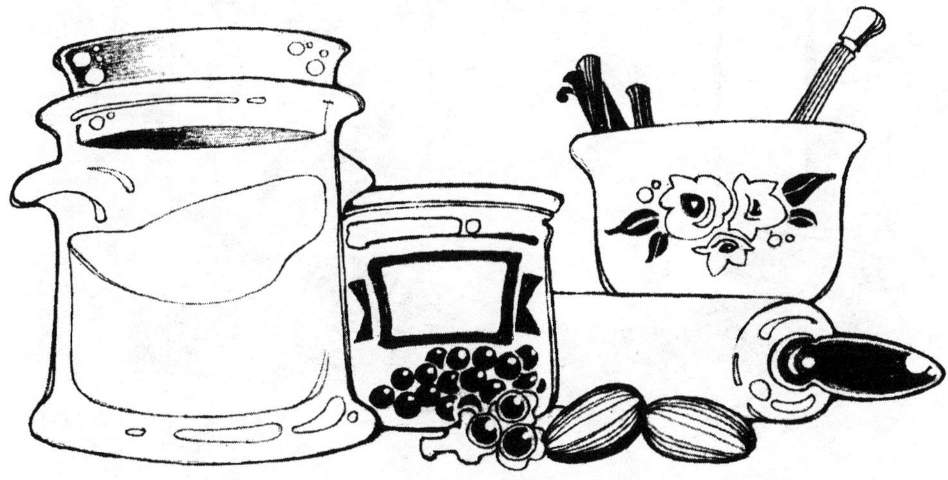

Elizabeth David's Spice Blend

This is a sweet, peppery spice blend, which makes a marvelous addition to breads. See Yeasted Spice Bread on page 30, and Hot Cross Buns on page 32.)

1 large nutmeg, grated
1 6-inch stick cinnamon
1 tablespoon white peppercorns or allspice berries
2 scant teaspoons, or about 30, cloves
1½ teaspoons dried ginger, or a piece about 2 inches long

Break up the cinnamon stick and grate the nutmeg. Place them, along with the other ingredients, in a spice mill and grind to a powder. Keep in a covered jar in a cool, dark place.

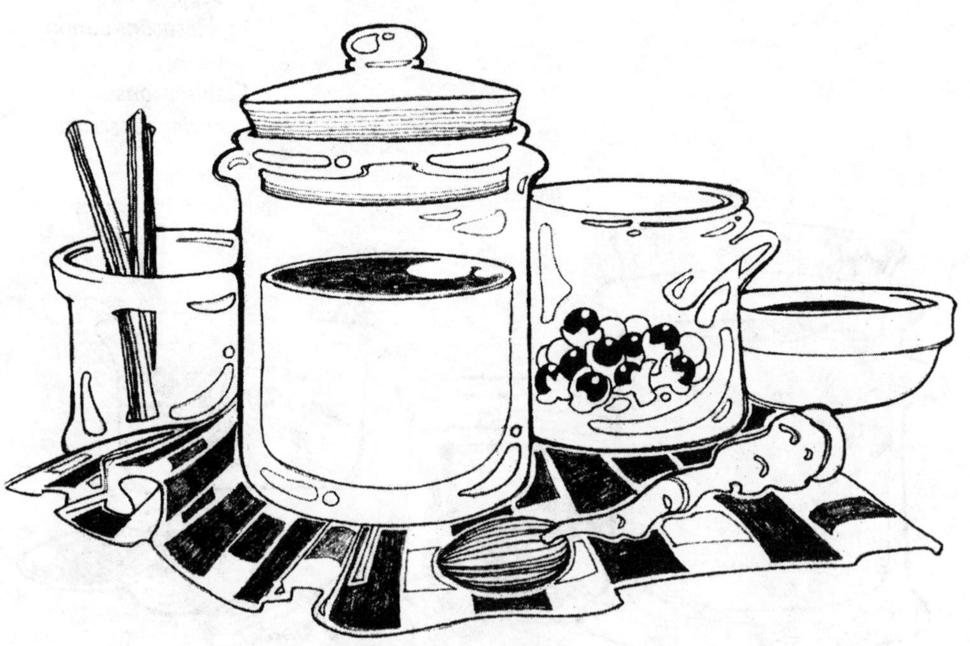

1
BREADS

BUCKWHEAT-SESAME CRACKERS WITH FENNEL

Makes 3 to 4 dozen

4 teaspoons fennel seeds
1½ cups whole wheat flour
¼ cup buckwheat flour
¼ cup sesame seeds
½ teaspoon sea salt
¼ cup safflower or vegetable oil
⅓ cup water

1. Preheat the oven to 350°F. Oil 2 cookie sheets.

2. Place the fennel seeds in a mortar and pestle and crack.

3. Mix together the flours, sesame seeds, salt, and cracked fennel seeds. Add the oil and cut in by taking the flour up by handfuls and rolling briskly between the palms of your hands. (This can also be done in a food processor.)

4. Add the water. The dough should have a pie crust consistency (though coarser). If too dry, add a little more water. Gather up the dough and roll out on a well-floured board or between pieces of waxed paper. Dough should be about ⅛ inch thick.

5. Cut into squares or use a cookie cutter. Place on the prepared baking sheets and bake in the preheated oven until brown, about 20 to 25 minutes, switching the positions of the baking sheets halfway through the baking. Don't let them get too brown or they'll taste bitter. Cool on racks.

Yeasted Spice Bread with Zucchini and Raisins

Makes 2 loaves

1 tablespoon active dry yeast
½ cup lukewarm water
½ cup lukewarm milk
¼ cup mild-flavored honey
1 egg
2 tablespoons melted butter
1 tablespoon Elizabeth David's Spice Blend (page 28)
1½ teaspoons salt
2 teaspoons grated orange rind
1½ cups shredded zucchini
¼ cup bran
3 cups whole wheat flour

1. Dissolve the yeast in the water. Add the milk and honey, and beat in the egg and butter. Stir in the spice mix, salt, grated orange rind, and zucchini. Fold in the bran and the cornmeal. Begin adding the flour (not including the additional unbleached white flour for kneading), a cup at a time, and fold in after each addition. When all the flour has been added, let the dough rest in the bowl for 15 minutes.

2. Turn out the dough on a well-floured work surface and knead for 10 minutes, or until the dough is smooth. Add flour as necessary. The dough is very moist, and it might be easier to knead by picking up the dough and throwing it against your floured work surface, rather than folding and leaning into the dough. Just take up the dough, slap it down on the table, take it up again, etc. This is also an effective way to develop the gluten.

3. Rinse, dry, and oil your bowl. Place the dough in it rounded side down first, then rounded side up. Cover and let rise in a warm place for 45 minutes to an hour, or until doubled in bulk.

4. Punch down the dough, turn out onto a floured surface, and knead in the raisins. Divide the dough in half and form into rounds or small loaves. Let rise on a greased baking sheet or in greased bread pans for 45 minutes to an hour, or until doubled.

5. Preheat the oven to 375°F. Slash the loaves and brush with water or egg. Bake 35 to 45 minutes, or until they sound hollow when tapped. Remove from the pans and cool on a rack.

1 cup stone-ground cornmeal
1 cup unbleached white flour plus up to 1 more cup additional for kneading
1 cup raisins
1 beaten egg, if desired, for brushing the loaves

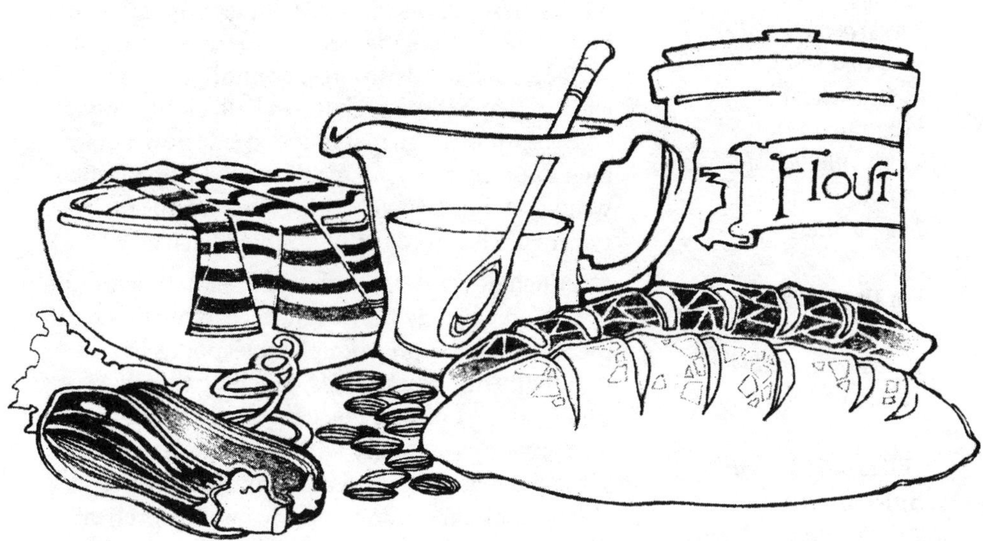

Hot Cross Buns

Makes 2 dozen

1 cup milk
1 tablespoon active dry yeast
¼ cup mild-flavored honey
4 tablespoons unsalted butter, melted and cooled
2 eggs
3 cups whole wheat pastry flour
1 teaspoon sea salt
2 teaspoons Elizabeth David's Spice Blend (see below)*
⅔ cup currants
1 cup unbleached white flour, as needed
1 egg white

For the Glaze:
2 tablespoons lemon juice
1 tablespoon mild-flavored honey

***Elizabeth David's Spice Blend:**
1 large nutmeg, grated
1 tablespoon white or black peppercorns or *allspice berries*
1 6-inch cinnamon stick
2 teaspoons (or about 30) cloves

1. Warm the milk to lukewarm in a small saucepan. Dissolve the yeast in the milk (making sure the milk is no hotter than lukewarm) and let sit 5 minutes. Then stir in the honey, melted butter, and beaten eggs.

2. Place 3 cups pastry flour in a large bowl and stir in the spice mix and the salt. Make a well in the center and pour in the milk mixture. Fold in the flour with a large wooden spoon. Add the currants and fold in. Dough will be quite wet.

3. Place ½ cup unbleached white flour on your work surface and scrape the dough out of the bowl. Knead, flouring your hands and the work surface, for 5 to 10 minutes, or until dough is elastic. Shape the dough into a ball, oil the bowl, and place the dough in it rounded side down first, then rounded side up. Cover the bowl with plastic wrap or a damp towel and set in a warm spot to rise for 1½ hours, or until doubled in size.

4. Punch down the dough and knead for a minute or two on a lightly floured surface. Now pinch off pieces of the dough, about 2 tablespoons in size, and shape into round balls, pinching together tightly at the bottom. Place on oiled baking sheets and press down gently with the bottom of a jar or glass. Cover and let rise until doubled in volume, about 45 minutes to an hour. Meanwhile preheat the oven to 375°F.

5. Beat the egg white until frothy and gently brush the tops of the buns. Using a very sharp knife or a razor blade, cut an X across the top of each bun. Place in the preheated oven and bake 20 minutes, or until lightly browned.

6. While the buns are baking, mix together the lemon juice and honey. As soon as you remove the buns from the oven, brush with the glaze mixture. Cool on racks. These are marvelous warm, with tea.

1½ teaspoons powdered ginger (⅛ ounce dried ginger root)

Combine all the ingredients and grind to a powder in a spice mill. Store in a well-sealed jar.

BOSTON BROWN BREAD WITH GINGER

This steamed dark bread is adapted from my version in The Vegetarian Feast. *I've spiced up the original version with ground ginger.*

Makes 2 loaves

1 cup rye flour
1 cup stone-ground yellow cornmeal
1 cup whole wheat flour
2 teaspoons baking soda
1 teaspoon sea salt
1 tablespoon ground ginger
¾ cup dark molasses
2 cups buttermilk or plain, low-fat yogurt
1 cup raisins

1. Sift together the rye flour, cornmeal, wheat flour, baking soda, ginger, and salt. Stir in the molasses and buttermilk or yogurt and blend well. Stir in the raisins.

2. Butter two 1-pound coffee or juice cans, or several smaller cans, generously. Fill each can three-quarters full of batter. Butter pieces of foil and cover the cans, sealing well with tape if necessary.

3. Place the cans in a large pot and pour in water to a depth of 2 inches. Bring the water to a boil, cover, and reduce heat to very low. Simmer for 3 hours, checking once in a while to make sure the water hasn't boiled off.

4. Remove the cans from the pot, unmold, and cool on a rack. If your bread seems too moist, place in a moderate oven for 10 minutes.

BLACK BREAD

Makes 2 large loaves

1 heaping tablespoon Postum dissolved in ½ cup hot water, or ½ cup strong coffee
2 tablespoons active dry yeast
2 cups lukewarm water
¼ cup dark molasses
1 teaspoon ground ginger
2 cups whole wheat breadcrumbs
2 cups unbleached white flour, plus more as necessary for kneading
4 tablespoons safflower oil
2 teaspoons sea salt
3 cups rye flour
2 cups whole wheat flour
1 egg, beaten with 3 tablespoons of water for egg wash
Poppy seeds for the topping

1. Allow Postum or coffee to cool to lukewarm.

2. In a large bowl, dissolve the yeast in the lukewarm water. Add the molasses and ginger and stir together. When the Postum or coffee has cooled to lukewarm, add it to the yeast mixture.

3. Add the breadcrumbs and unbleached flour, a cup at a time, and stir 100 times. Set this sponge aside in a warm place, covered with plastic wrap or a damp towel, to rise for 50 to 60 minutes.

4. Fold in the oil and sea salt. Add the rye flour a cup at a time, and fold in. Begin adding the whole wheat flour. After 1 cup you should be able to turn out the dough, which will be sticky, onto your kneading surface. Place the other cup of whole wheat flour on your kneading surface, scrape out the dough, and begin to knead. Knead for 10 minutes, adding unbleached white flour as necessary.

5. When the dough is stiff and elastic, shape into a ball. Oil the bowl, then place the dough in it seam side down first, then seam side up. Cover and let rise in a warm place until doubled in bulk, about 1½ hours.

6. Punch down the dough and turn it out onto a lightly floured board. Divide into two equal pieces and shape the pieces into two long or round loaves. Make the loaves high, as the dough will spread out. Brush with oil and place on oiled cookie sheets or in baguette pans. Cover with a damp towel and let rise again for 30 minutes, or until nearly doubled in bulk.

7. Preheat the oven to 400°F. Brush the loaves with the egg wash and sprinkle with poppy seeds. Brush once more, slash, and place in the preheated oven. Bake 40 to 45 minutes, brushing again with the egg wash halfway through the baking.

8. Remove from the baking sheet or pans and let cool on a rack.

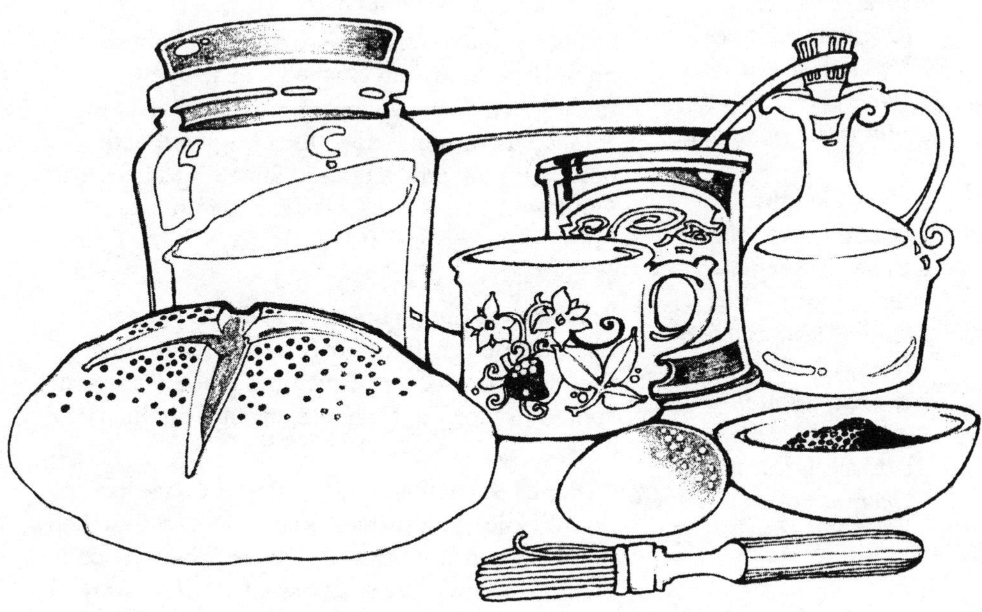

Buckwheat and Whole Wheat Bread with Cumin

Makes 2 loaves

For the Sponge:
1 tablespoon active dry yeast
2 cups lukewarm water
1 cup plain, low-fat yogurt
2 tablespoons honey
1 tablespoon molasses
2 cups unbleached white flour
2 cups whole wheat flour

For the Dough:
1 tablespoon sea salt
4 tablespoons safflower oil
2 heaping tablespoons cumin seeds
1 cup buckwheat flour
¾ cup cracked wheat
3 cups whole wheat flour, more as needed
1 egg, for egg wash

1. First make the sponge. Dissolve the yeast in the lukewarm water and add the honey and molasses. Stir in the yogurt, then the flours, a cup at a time. When all 4 cups have been added, stir 100 times. Cover with plastic wrap or a damp towel and set in a warm place to rise for an hour, after which time it should be bubbly.

2. Fold in the sea salt and oil, then the cumin, buckwheat flour, and cracked wheat. Begin folding in the whole wheat flour, a cup at a time. As soon as you can scrape the dough out of the bowl, turn out onto a floured kneading surface. Flour your hands and knead for 10 minutes, or until the dough is stiff and elastic, adding flour as necessary.

3. Shape the dough into a ball and oil your bowl. Place the dough in the bowl, seam side up first, then seam side down. Cover and place in a warm spot to rise for 1 to 1½ hours, or until doubled in bulk.

4. Punch down the dough and turn out onto a floured kneading surface. Knead a few times, then divide in two and form two loaves. Place in oiled bread pans and cover. Let rise 40 minutes to an hour, or until they rise above the tops of the pans.

5. Ten to fifteen minutes before the end of the rising time, preheat the oven to 375°F. Gently brush the tops of the loaves with beaten egg, slash with a razor blade or sharp knife, and place in the preheated oven.

6. Bake 50 to 60 minutes, or until golden brown and the loaves respond to tapping with a hollow, thumping sound. Remove from the pans and cool on a rack.

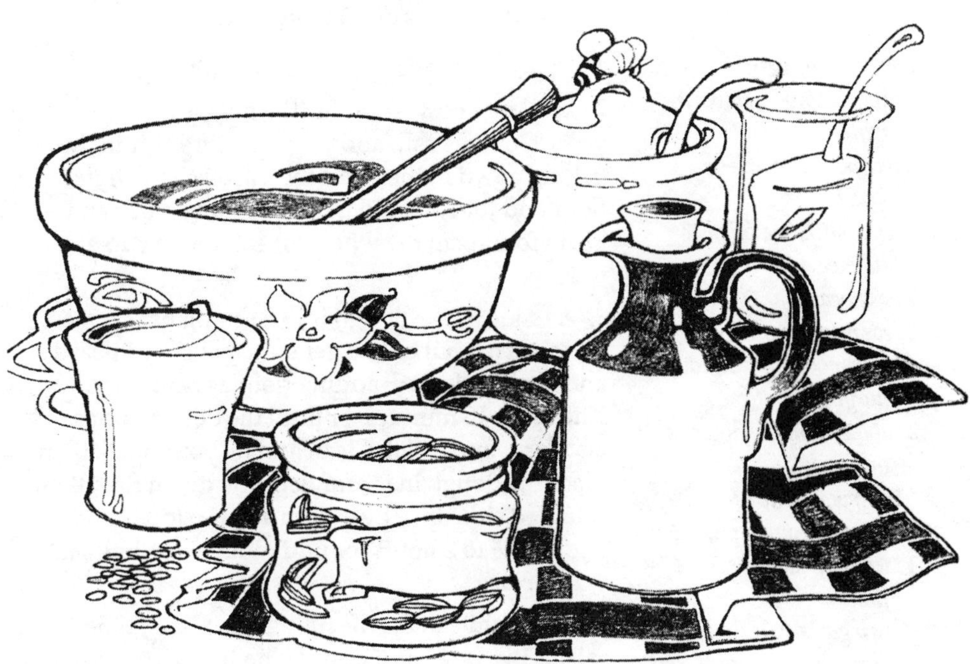

NAANS WITH SWEET PINE NUT–RAISIN FILLING

Naans are flat, yeasted breads which are traditionally baked in a Tandoori oven but still yield delicious results when baked under a broiler. These naans are stuffed with a sweet, anisy paste made with golden raisins, pine nuts, and spices. Some of the paste is spread in the middle and some on the top. They are great for breakfast as well as lunch or dinner.

Makes 6 large naans

For the Dough:
2 tablespoons lukewarm water
2 teaspoons active dry yeast
¾ cup milk, warmed to lukewarm
1 egg, beaten
2 teaspoons honey
4 tablespoons plain, low-fat yogurt
2 tablespoons safflower oil
1 teaspoon baking powder (optional)
1 cup unbleached white flour
½ cup garbanzo flour
3 cups whole wheat flour
Additional flour for dusting

For the Filling:
1½ cups golden raisins
½ cup pine nuts

1. Dissolve the yeast in the water in a cup.

2. In a large bowl combine the milk, egg, honey, yogurt, oil, sea salt, and yeast mixture. Stir in the baking powder, then add the unbleached white flour and fold in. Fold in the garbanzo flour and begin folding in the whole wheat flour a cup at a time.

3. As soon as the dough is in a semblance of one piece, turn it out onto a generously floured board and begin to knead, adding flour as necessary. Knead for 10 minutes, or until the dough is elastic, and form into a ball. Clean and oil your bowl, then place the dough in it rounded side down first, then rounded side up. Cover with a damp towel and let rise for 1½ to 2 hours, or until doubled in bulk, in a warm place.

4. Meanwhile make the filling. Place the golden raisins in a bowl and pour on boiling water to cover. Let plump 15 minutes, then drain and pat dry with paper towels. Blend to a paste in a food processor or mash in a mortar and pestle. Add the pine nuts and spices and continue to mash together, but make sure the pine nuts retain some texture. Some can remain whole.

5. When the dough has risen, preheat the broiler. Brush three baking sheets with oil.

6. Punch down the dough and turn out onto a lightly floured work surface. Knead a few times, then divide into six equal pieces. Shape these into balls, then roll each one out to a teardrop shape so that they taper at the bottom and are about ¼ inch thick. Spread with 1 heaped tablespoon of the pine nut–raisin paste (there will be some left over, which you will spread on the top) and fold the narrow bottom half of the dough up over the top half. Fold the overlapping edges in and over and pinch together tightly. Place on the baking sheets, two on a sheet, cover with a damp towel, and let rise 20 minutes.

7. These bake very quickly under the broiler, and you have to watch them carefully. Place about 3 inches from the broiler and let bake for 1 minute. Check after 1 minute and if they aren't beginning to brown continue baking for a second minute. If they are beginning to brown, reduce heat slightly for the second minute. After 2 minutes they should be golden brown (leave in, watching carefully, up to another minute if they are not). Turn and cook for 1 minute on the other side. Now spread some of the remaining pine nut–raisin paste over the top of each naan and place under the broiler for another minute or two. Remove from the heat and serve hot. These can be reheated in the oven, wrapped in foil, and will keep several days in the refrigerator. You can also roll out the naans and keep the dough refrigerated, covered with plastic wrap, for up to a day.

1¼ teaspoons crushed anise seeds
½ teaspoon crushed cardamom seeds
½ cup plain low-fat yogurt

Naans with Spicy Chick Pea (Garbanzo) Filling

These naans are almost like pita bread with the stuffing baked right inside. They are a high-protein meal in themselves.

Makes 6 large naans

For the Dough:
2 tablespoons lukewarm water
2 teaspoons active dry yeast
¾ cup milk, warmed to lukewarm
1 egg, beaten
2 teaspoons honey
4 tablespoons plain, low-fat yogurt
2 tablespoons safflower oil
1 teaspoon sea salt
1 teaspoon baking powder (optional)
1 cup unbleached white flour
½ cup garbanzo flour
3 cups whole wheat flour
Additional flour for dusting

For the Filling:
2 cups garbanzos, cooked
½ cup plain, low-fat yogurt
1 teaspoon crushed cumin seeds
1 teaspoon crushed fennel seeds

1. Dissolve the yeast in the water in a cup.

2. In a large bowl combine the milk, egg, honey, yogurt, oil, sea salt, and yeast mixture. Stir in the baking powder, then add the unbleached white flour and fold in. Fold in the garbanzo flour and begin folding in the whole wheat flour a cup at a time.

3. As soon as the dough is in a semblance of one piece, turn it out onto a generously floured board and begin to knead, adding flour as necessary. Knead for 10 minutes, or until the dough is elastic, and form into a ball. Clean and oil your bowl, then place the dough in it rounded side down first, then rounded side up. Cover with a damp towel and let rise for 1½ to 2 hours, or until doubled in bulk, in a warm place.

4. Meanwhile make the filling. Mash the garbanzos with a mortar and pestle, or in a food processor or blender, and mix with the yogurt and spices, which you have crushed with a mortar and pestle or in a spice mill. Season to taste with sea salt, cayenne, and freshly ground pepper. It should be a little piquant and should have a pastelike consistency.

5. When the dough has risen, preheat the broiler. Brush three baking sheets with oil.

6. Punch down the dough and turn out onto a lightly floured work surface. Knead a few times, then divide into six equal pieces. Shape these into balls, then roll each one out to a teardrop shape so

that they taper at the bottom and are about ¼ inch thick. Spread with 3 heaping tablespoons of the garbanzo paste and fold the narrow bottom half of the dough up over the top half. Fold the overlapping edges in and over and pinch together tightly. Place on the baking sheets, two on a sheet, cover with a damp towel, and let rise 20 minutes.

7. These bake very quickly under the broiler, and you have to watch them carefully. Place about 3 inches from the broiler and let bake for 1 minute. Check after 1 minute, and if they aren't beginning to brown, continue baking for a second minute. If they are beginning to brown, reduce heat slightly for the second minute. After 2 minutes they should be golden brown (leave, watching carefully, up to another minute if they are not). Turn and repeat this process on the other side. Remove from the heat and serve hot. These can be reheated in the oven, wrapped in foil, and will keep several days in the refrigerator. You can also roll out the naans and keep the dough refrigerated, covered with plastic wrap, for up to a day.

These are large and filling and can be cut in half to serve or can even be cut into pieces to serve as hors d'oeuvres. The protein is complete, and they make a good main dish.

1 teaspoon crushed cardamom seeds
⅛ teaspoon cayenne pepper, or more to taste
Sea salt and freshly ground pepper to taste

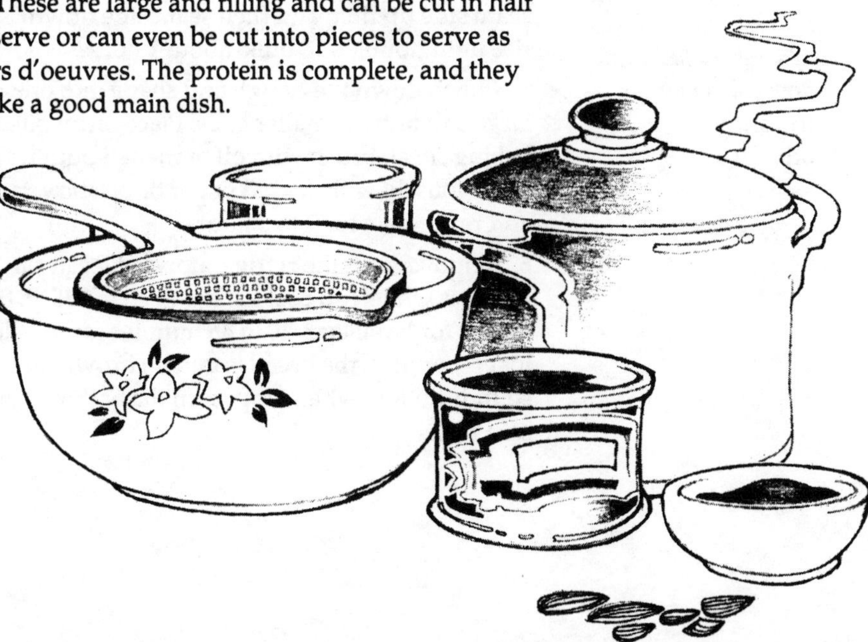

Swedish Limpa

This sweet, subtly spiced bread is adapted from James Beard's recipe.

Makes 1 large, round loaf

1 tablespoon active dry yeast
4 tablespoons lukewarm water
2 cups dark beer, heated to lukewarm
6 tablespoons honey
2 tablespoons melted butter or safflower oil
2 teaspoons sea salt
1 teaspoon ground cardamom
1 teaspoon crushed anise seeds
2 tablespoons grated orange peel
2½ cups rye flour
1 cup whole wheat flour
2 cups unbleached white flour, plus more as necessary for kneading

1. Dissolve the yeast in the water in a large bowl and let sit for 5 minutes. Add the beer, honey, melted butter or oil, sea salt, cardamom, anise seeds, and orange peel and mix together well.

2. Mix together the flours and fold 3 cups into the yeast mixture. Stir 100 times, cover with plastic wrap or a damp towel, and set this sponge in a warm place for 1 hour.

3. Stir down the sponge and fold in a cup of the flour. Continue to add flour until you can turn out the dough, which will be sticky, onto a floured kneading surface. Knead for 10 to 15 minutes, adding only enough flour to make the dough workable. When the dough is stiff, form into a ball.

4. Rinse the bowl, oil it and place the dough in it seam side up first, and then seam side down. Let rise until doubled in bulk, about 1 hour.

5. Punch down the dough and shape into one large ball or two smaller balls. Place on an oiled baking sheet, brush with oil or melted butter, cover loosely with waxed paper or plastic wrap, and refrigerate for 2 to 3 hours.

6. Remove from the refrigerator and let sit for 15 minutes while you preheat the oven to 375°F. Bake 1 hour for large loaf, 40 to 45 minutes for smaller loaves, or until the bread is golden brown and sounds hollow when tapped on the bottom. Cool on a rack.

Cheese and Mustard Bread

This bread is like a cheese sandwich with the cheese and mustard baked right into the loaf. When you toast it, the fragrance of the mustard and cheese emerges, and it smells like a grilled cheese sandwich. You can reduce the mustard by half if you want a more subtle flavor. This bread freezes well.

Makes 1 loaf

1 tablespoon active dry yeast
½ cup lukewarm water
½ cup lukewarm milk
1 tablespoon mild-flavored honey
1 teaspoon sea salt
1 teaspoon freshly ground black pepper
1 egg, lightly beaten
1 teaspoon crushed rosemary
½ cup Dijon-style mustard
1 tablespoon grated onion
4 ounces grated sharp Cheddar cheese
3 cups whole wheat flour
Up to ½ cup unbleached white flour for kneading
1 egg, beaten with 4 tablespoons water, for egg wash

1. Dissolve the yeast in the water and let sit for 10 minutes. Add the milk, honey, sea salt, pepper, egg, rosemary, mustard, and onion and beat well. Stir in the grated cheese.

2. Fold in the whole wheat flour a cup at a time. When the dough comes away from the sides of the bowl, place a half cup of flour on your kneading surface and turn out the dough. Knead for 10 minutes, or until the dough is smooth and elastic. Add more flour as necessary.

3. Oil the bowl and place the dough in it seam side up first, then seam side down. Let rise in a warm place for 30 minutes.

4. Punch the dough down, knead a few times, and form into a loaf. Butter a loaf pan and place the dough in it, seam side up first, then seam side down. Cover loosely with plastic wrap and refrigerate overnight.

5. In the morning remove the dough from the refrigerator. Let it stand in a warm place for 45 minutes.

6. Preheat the oven to 350°F. Brush the loaf with egg wash, slash the top, and bake in the preheated oven for 50 minutes. Remove from the pan and cool on a rack.

BANANA NUT BREAD

Makes 1 loaf

1 cup whole wheat flour
1 cup unbleached white flour
1 teaspoon baking soda
1 teaspoon cinnamon
½ teaspoon nutmeg
½ teaspoon sea salt
4 tablespoons melted butter
½ cup mild-flavored honey
1 teaspoon vanilla extract
2 eggs
3 medium-sized bananas, mashed
4 tablespoons plain, low-fat yogurt
1 cup chopped walnuts

1. Preheat the oven to 375°F. Butter an 8 x 5 x 3 inch loaf pan.

2. Sift together the flours, baking soda, spices, and sea salt.

3. Beat together the melted butter, honey, vanilla, eggs, bananas, and yogurt.

4. Quickly stir the wet ingredients into the dry (or vice versa). Fold in the chopped nuts. Turn into the prepared bread pan and bake in the preheated oven for 50 to 60 minutes, or until a cake tester comes out clean.

5. Remove from the oven and let cool in the pan for 10 minutes, then turn out onto a rack and cool completely.

Zucchini Bread

Makes 1 loaf

1. Preheat the oven to 350°F. Butter a 9 x 5 inch loaf pan.

2. Beat together the eggs, oil, honey, and vanilla. Stir in zucchini and orange rind.

3. Sift together the flour, baking soda, baking powder, sea salt, and spices. Stir into liquid mixture and mix just until well blended. Fold in the nuts.

4. Pour into the prepared bread pan and bake in the preheated oven on the middle rack for 1 hour and 15 minutes, or until a tester comes out clean.

5. Cool for 10 minutes in the pans, then reverse on a rack and cool completely. Wrap in plastic wrap and foil and let sit overnight so the flavors will develop. This makes a very nice tea or dessert bread.

4 eggs
¾ cup safflower or vegetable oil
¾ cup mild-flavored honey
2 teaspoons vanilla extract
1 tablespoon grated orange rind
2 cups (½ pound) grated zucchini
2 cups whole wheat pastry flour
2 teaspoons baking soda
1 teaspoon baking powder
½ teaspoon sea salt
2 teaspoons ground cinnamon
1 teaspoon ground cloves
1 teaspoon ground nutmeg
½ teaspoon ground allspice
1 cup shelled walnuts or pecans, chopped

Pain D'Epices

This recipe is from my Herbs and Honey Cookery. *I can't leave it out of this collection of spice recipes. There are many versions of this bread, and this is just one of them.*

Makes 1 loaf

4 ounces unsalted butter or safflower oil
6 tablespoons strong-flavored honey
2 tablespoons molasses
¾ cup milk
1 egg, beaten
1 tablespoon lemon juice
2 cups whole wheat flour
½ cup rye flour
1 teaspoon baking soda
1½ tablespoons ground anise seeds
¼ teaspoon ground allspice
½ teaspoon ground cardamom
½ teaspoon ground coriander
½ teaspoon grated nutmeg
¼ teaspoon ground ginger
¼ teaspoon ground cloves
Pinch of sea salt

1. Preheat the oven to 375°F.

2. Cream together the butter or safflower oil, the honey, and the molasses. Beat in the milk, egg, and lemon juice.

3. Sift together the flours, soda, sea salt, and spices. Stir into the liquid mixture and blend well.

4. Butter a loaf pan and line with buttered waxed paper. Spoon in the batter and bake in the preheated oven for 50 to 60 minutes, or until a tester comes out clean. Turn out onto a wire rack and remove the paper. Cool completely and wrap tightly in plastic wrap and foil. Let sit for several days before eating so that the spices can ripen. This will stay good for 2 weeks.

Cheese, Pepper, and Mustard Muffins

Makes 12 to 14 muffin

1. Preheat the oven to 375°F. Butter muffin tins.
2. Sift together the flours, salt, pepper, and baking powder.
3. Beat together the eggs, oil or melted butter, honey, milk, and mustard. Stir in the cheese.
4. Quickly stir the wet ingredients into the dry and spoon into muffin tins. Bake 20 minutes in the preheated oven. Serve hot, or cool on racks.

1 cup whole wheat flour
1 cup unbleached white flour
½ teaspoon sea salt
2½ teaspoons baking powder
2 teaspoons freshly ground black pepper
2 eggs
¼ cup safflower oil or melted butter
2 teaspoons mild-flavored honey
1 cup milk
2 tablespoons Dijon-style mustard
1 cup grated Cheddar or Monterey jack cheese

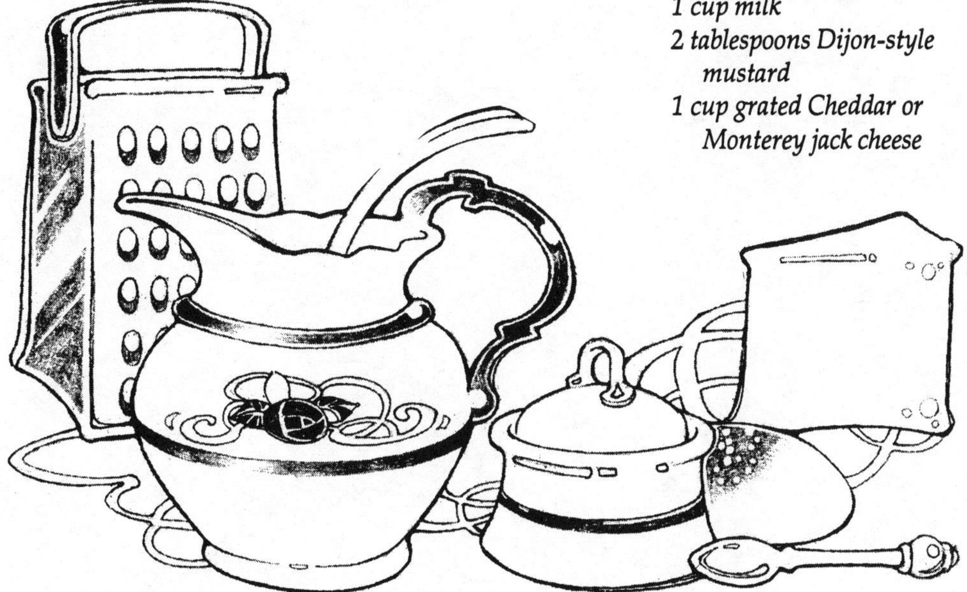

Jalapeño Corn Muffins

Makes 15 muffins

1¼ cups stone-ground yellow cornmeal
¾ cup whole wheat flour
2½ teaspoons baking powder
½ teaspoon sea salt
1 egg
4 tablespoons safflower oil or melted butter
1 tablespoon mild-flavored honey
1½ cups milk
1 to 2 jalapeño chili peppers, to taste, seeded and chopped

1. Preheat the oven to 400°F. Butter muffin tins.

2. Sift together the cornmeal, flour, baking powder, and sea salt.

3. In another bowl beat together the egg, oil or melted butter, honey, and milk. Stir in the chopped jalapeños.

4. Quickly stir the wet ingredients into the dry, being careful not to stir too much. Spoon into muffin tins (this is a runny batter) and bake in a preheated oven for 20 minutes, or until firm and beginning to brown. Serve hot, or cool on racks.

SWEET POTATO MUFFINS

Makes 16 muffins

1 cup unbleached white flour
1 cup whole wheat flour
1 tablespoon baking powder
1 teaspoon cinnamon
½ teaspoon grated nutmeg
¼ teaspoon sea salt
¾ pound cooked, mashed sweet potatoes
4 tablespoons melted butter
½ cup apple juice
½ cup mild-flavored honey
4 tablespoons fresh lime juice
3 eggs
½ cup milk or plain, low-fat yogurt

1. Preheat the oven to 400°F. Butter muffin tins.

2. Sift together the flours, baking powder, sea salt, and spices.

3. Beat together the sweet potatoes, melted butter, apple juice, honey, lime juice, eggs, and milk or yogurt. Quickly stir into the dry ingredients. Spoon into muffin tins and bake for 25 to 30 minutes, or until beginning to brown. Cool on a rack or serve warm.

Pecan Rolls

Makes 2 dozen

1 cup raisins
Boiling water to cover the raisins
1 cup soy or cow's milk, scalded and cooled to lukewarm
1 cup lukewarm orange juice
1 tablespoon active dry yeast
6 tablespoons mild-flavored honey
6 tablespoons safflower oil or melted butter
½ cup plain, low-fat yogurt
2 tablespoons grated orange peel
1 teaspoon sea salt
1 teaspoon ground cardamom
½ teaspoon ground mace or nutmeg
4 tablespoons soy flour
2 cups unbleached white flour
3 cups whole wheat flour, or as needed
4 tablespoons additional melted butter
2 tablespoons additional honey
1½ cups chopped pecans
Cinnamon

1. Soak the raisins in boiling water to cover for 15 minutes and then drain.

2. Dissolve the yeast in the milk and add the orange juice and honey. Let sit about 10 minutes.

3. Stir in the 6 tablespoons safflower oil or melted butter, raisins, yogurt, orange peel, sea salt, spices, and soy flour. Mix well and fold in the unbleached white flour, a cup at a time. Begin folding in the whole wheat flour, and when the dough comes away from the sides of the bowl, turn it out onto a floured surface. Dough will be sticky.

4. Knead 10 to 15 minutes, adding flour as necessary to the kneading surface. Shape into a ball.

5. Clean the bowl and oil it. Place the dough in it seam side down, then seam side up. Cover with plastic wrap or a damp towel and let the dough rise in a warm place for 1½ to 2 hours, or until double in bulk.

6. Punch down the dough, knead a few times, and cut in two. Roll out each half into a large rectangle about ¼ inch thick.

7. Melt the additional 4 tablespoons butter and the 2 tablespoons honey together over low heat. Brush the rectangles with this mixture and sprinkle generously with cinnamon. Spread ¾ cup of pecans evenly over each rectangle, and roll up lengthwise tightly like a jelly roll.

8. Cut each cylinder into rolls 1½ inches thick. Butter muffin tins.

9. Melt together the butter and honey for the topping, and add the cinnamon. Brush the muffin tins with this mixture and sprinkle with a few

chopped pecans. Place the cut pecan rolls in the tins. Cover loosely with plastic wrap and let rise 30 minutes, then refrigerate overnight. Retain the remaining butter/honey mixture for the completed rolls.

10. In the morning, preheat the oven to 350° F. and remove the rolls from the refrigerator. Let sit in a warm place for 30 minutes, then bake for 20 to 25 minutes, or until brown, in the pre-heated oven. Meanwhile heat the remaining butter/honey mixture.

11. Remove the pecan rolls from the oven, reverse onto a rack, brush the tops with the remaining butter and honey, and allow to cool.

For the Topping:

⅓ cup butter, melted
¼ cup honey, warmed with the butter
½ teaspoon cinnamon
½ cup chopped pecans

Yogurt Coffee Cake with Apple-Nut Filling

4 tablespoons unsalted butter
4 tablespoons safflower oil
¾ cup mild-flavored honey
3 eggs, beaten
1½ cups plain, low-fat yogurt
1 tablespoon vanilla extract
1 cup whole wheat pastry flour
1 cup unbleached white flour
1 tablespoon baking powder
1 teaspoon cinnamon
¼ teaspoon sea salt

For the Filling:
3 medium-sized apples, peeled, cored, and thinly sliced
2 tablespoons lemon juice
1 tablespoon cinnamon
½ teaspoon ground nutmeg
½ teaspoon ground cloves
¾ cup chopped pecans or walnuts

1. Pregeat the oven to 350°F. Butter a 2-quart rectangular baking dish or a 12-inch cake pan.

2. Cream together the butter, oil, and honey. Beat in the eggs, yogurt, and vanilla.

3. Sift together the flours, baking powder, cinnamon, and sea salt. Fold into the wet ingredients. Stir together until just blended. Do not overbeat.

4. Toss the thinly sliced apples with the lemon juice, spices, and chopped nuts.

5. Turn half the batter into the prepared pan. Layer the filling evenly over the batter. Top with the remaining batter.

6. Place in the preheated oven and bake 60 to 90 minutes, or until a tester when inserted in the middle comes out clean. Remove from the oven and cool on a rack for 30 minutes, then cut in wedges or squares and serve.

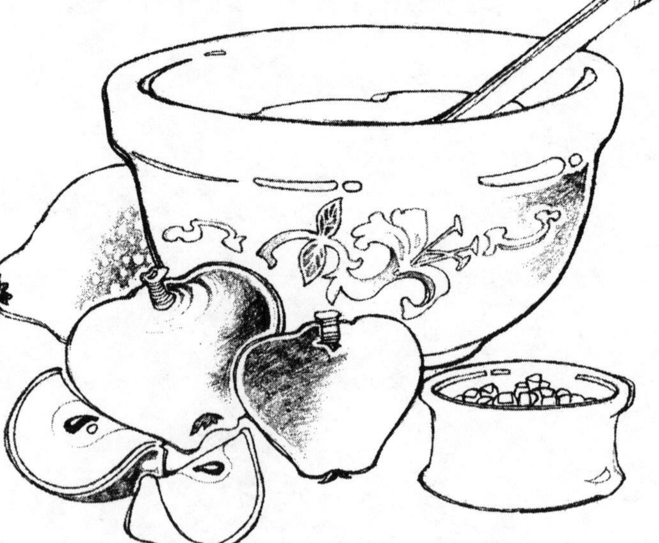

PECAN-YOGURT COFFEE CAKE

4 tablespoons unsalted butter
4 tablespoons safflower oil
¾ cup mild-flavored honey
3 eggs, beaten
1½ cups plain, low-fat yogurt
1 tablespoon vanilla extract
1 cup whole wheat pastry flour
1 cup unbleached white flour
1 tablespoon baking powder
¼ teaspoon sea salt

For the Filling:
2 cups chopped pecans or walnuts
⅓ cup raisins (optional)
1 tablespoon cinnamon
½ teaspoon ground nutmeg
½ teaspoon ground cloves

1. Preheat the oven to 350°F. Butter a 2-quart rectangular baking dish or a 12-inch cake pan.

2. Cream together the butter, oil, and honey. Beat in the eggs, yogurt, and vanilla. Sift together the flours, baking powder, and sea salt. Fold into the wet ingredients. Stir together until just blended. Do not overbeat. Mix together the nuts, optional raisins, and spices.

3. Turn half the batter into the prepared pan. Sprinkle the chopped nut-and-spice mixture in an even layer over the batter. Top with the remaining batter.

4. Place in the preheated oven and bake 60 to 90 minutes, or until a tester when inserted in the middle comes out clean. Remove from the oven and cool on a rack for 30 minutes, then cut in wedges or squares and serve.

2
SOUPS

VEGETABLE STOCK

Makes 2 quarts

2 quarts water
2 onions, quartered
Cloves from 1 head garlic, peeled
2 carrots, coarsely sliced
2 leeks, white part only, cleaned and coarsely sliced
4 potatoes, scrubbed and quartered
2 turnips, peeled and diced
2 stalks celery, coarsely sliced
2 sprigs parsley
1 bay leaf
¼ teaspoon thyme
Sea salt to taste

Combine all the ingredients in a soup pot and bring to a simmer. Cover, reduce heat, and simmer 1 to 2 hours. Strain and discard the vegetables. This can be frozen and will last for several days in the refrigerator.

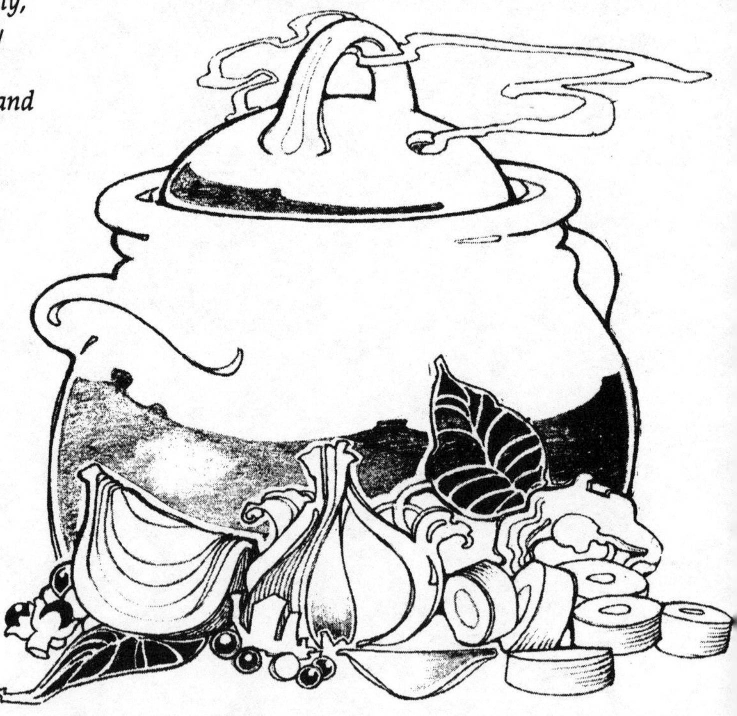

Easy Vegetable Bouillon

Makes 2 quarts

2 quarts water
4 vegetable bouillon cubes (available in natural food stores)
4 tablespoons soy sauce (more to taste)

Simmer the above ingredients together until the bouillon cubes dissolve.

Ginger-Vegetable Stock

Makes 2 quarts

2 quarts water
2 onions, quartered
Cloves from 1 head garlic, peeled
A 1-inch piece of ginger, peeled and thinly sliced
2 carrots, coarsely sliced
2 leeks, white part only, cleaned and coarsely sliced
4 potatoes, scrubbed and quartered
2 turnips, peeled and diced
2 stalks celery, coarsely sliced
2 sprigs parsley
1 bay leaf
¼ teaspoon thyme
Sea salt to taste
12 black peppercorns
4 whole cloves

Combine all the ingredients in a soup pot and bring to a simmer. Cover, reduce heat, and simmer 1 to 2 hours. Strain and discard the vegetables. This can be frozen and will last for several days in the refrigerator.

Cream of Spinach Soup

Serves 4 to 6

1 tablespoon safflower or vegetable oil
1 medium-sized onion, chopped
2 cloves garlic, minced or put through a press
1 teaspoon ground cumin
¼ teaspoon ground cloves
¼ teaspoon ground nutmeg
¼ teaspoon freshly ground pepper
3 cups regular or ginger-vegetable stock or bouillon (pages 54 and 55)
2 slices peeled, fresh ginger, about 1/8 inch thick
2 pounds fresh spinach, stemmed and washed, or 3 10-ounce packages, frozen, thawed
½ cup cooked rice, or 1 medium potato, peeled and diced
Sea salt to taste
1 cup milk
2 to 3 tablespoons heavy cream (to taste)
Juice of 1 lemon, or more, to taste
Additional pepper or cayenne pepper to taste
1 lemon, sliced, for garnish
Plain, low-fat yogurt for garnish

1. Heat the oil in a large, heavy-bottomed casserole or Dutch oven and sauté the onion with the garlic until translucent.

2. Add the spices and sauté 15 to 30 seconds, stirring.

3. Add the stock, spinach, ginger, and rice or potato and bring to a simmer. If using cooked rice, simmer 10 minutes, covered. If using potato, simmer 20 minutes, or until the potato is tender.

4. Remove from the heat and purée in a blender or put through the fine blade of a food mill.

5. Return to the pot, add the milk and cream, and add sea salt to taste. Heat through, stirring. Adjust seasonings, adding more spices if you wish.

6. Just before serving, stir in the lemon juice. Serve garnished with thin slices of lemon and a dollop of yogurt.

Note: This soup is also nice cold. In this case, chill before you add the lemon juice. Stir in the lemon juice just before serving.

Creamy Celery and Potato Soup with Lime

Serves 8

1. Tie the cinnamon stick, cloves, cardamom, and peppercorns loosely in a 6-inch square piece of cheesecloth. Using a rolling pin, pound the packet lightly to break up the spices.

2. Heat the oil in a large, heavy-bottomed soup pot or casserole and sauté the onion until tender. Add the garlic, ginger, celery, potato, and turmeric and sauté another couple of minutes, stirring. Add the vegetable stock and the spices in their cheesecloth bag and bring to a boil.

3. Reduce heat, cover, and simmer 30 minutes. Remove the cheesecloth bag and purée the soup in a blender or through a food mill.

4. Return the soup to the pot and add the milk. Heat through, add sea salt to taste, and stir in the coriander (alternatively, you can blend the coriander with the soup when you purée it). Stir in the lime juice and serve at once, garnishing with thin slices of lime.

1 cinnamon stick, 3 inches long, broken into pieces
6 whole cloves
3 white or green cardamom pods
1 teaspoon black peppercorns
1 tablespoon safflower or vegetable oil
2 medium onions, chopped
1 large clove garlic, peeled and left whole
2 teaspoons chopped fresh ginger
1 pound celery, chopped, with leaves
¾ pound potatoes, peeled and diced
¼ teaspoon turmeric
6 cups regular or ginger-vegetable stock (pages 54 and 55)
¾ cup milk
Sea salt to taste
¼ cup firmly packed coriander leaves, minced
Juice of 1 large lime (more to taste)
1 lime, sliced thin, for garnish

MULLIGATAWNY I

Serves 6 to 8

2 tablespoons safflower or vegetable oil, or butter
1 tablespoon curry powder
1 onion, minced
2 teaspoons minced fresh ginger
2 tart apples, peeled and diced
2 carrots, minced
½ cup raw peanuts
2 green peppers, seeded and chopped
2 quarts regular or ginger-vegetable stock (pages 54 and 55) or water
4 whole cloves
½ cup almonds, coarsely ground in a blender
1 tablespoon mild-flavored honey
2 tablespoons shredded coconut
½ cup raisins
1 teaspoon ground mace or nutmeg
Sea salt and freshly ground pepper to taste
3 tomatoes, peeled and chopped
1½ cups cooked long-grain brown rice
1 additional apple, sliced thin, for garnish

1. Heat the oil or butter in a large, heavy-bottomed soup pot or casserole and sauté the onion with the curry powder, fresh ginger, apples, carrots, peanuts, and green peppers for about 3 minutes, or until the onion begins to soften.

2. Add the vegetable stock or water, cloves, almonds, honey, coconut, raisins, mace or nutmeg, sea salt, pepper, and tomatoes and bring to a simmer. Cover and simmer over low heat for 30 minutes.

3. Remove half the soup and purée in a blender. Return to the pot and stir together well.

4. Heat through, adjust seasonings, and stir in the cooked brown rice. Serve, topping each bowl with thinly sliced apple.

MULLIGATAWNY II

Serves 6 to 8

1 onion, finely chopped
2 carrots, finely chopped
2 stalks celery, finely chopped
1 cup chopped mushrooms
1 pound eggplant, peeled and diced
2 turnips, chopped
2 slices peeled ginger root
6 cups regular vegetable stock (page 54)
2 large cloves garlic, peeled, left whole
2 sprigs coriander
¼ teaspoon ground black pepper
2 teaspoons curry powder, plus more to taste
Sea salt to taste
1 cup plain low-fat yogurt
3 tablespoons minced fresh coriander

1. Combine all the vegetables, ginger root, stock, two sprigs coriander, curry powder, and ground black pepper and bring to a simmer. Simmer 1 hour, covered.

2. Purée the soup in a blender or through a food mill. Return to the pot and adjust seasonings, adding salt to taste.

3. Heat through, and just before serving whisk in the yogurt and minced fresh coriander.

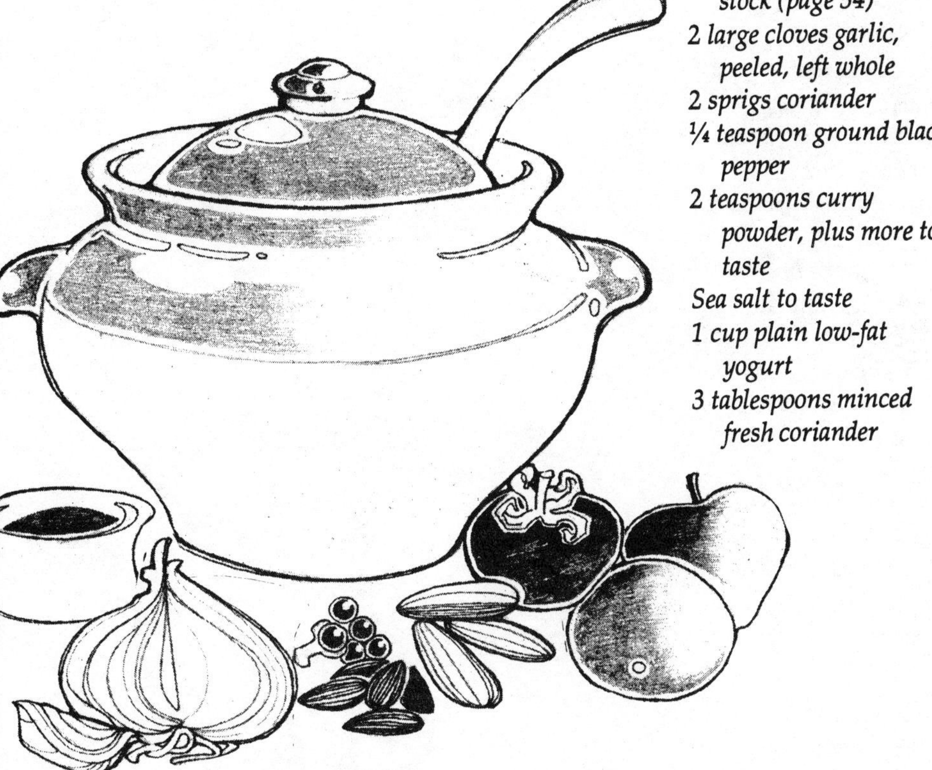

Spicy Apple Soup

Serves 6 to 8

1½ quarts water
2 pounds tart apples, peeled, cored, and sliced
1 cup dark or golden raisins
1½ teaspoons freshly grated nutmeg
2 teaspoons ground cinnamon
¼ to ½ teaspoon ground cloves, to taste
½ teaspoon ground allspice
3 to 4 tablespoons mild-flavored honey
½ cup rolled or flaked oats
Juice of ½ to 1 lemon, to taste
2 tablespoons brandy
1 cup plain low-fat yogurt
Thin slices of lemon and additional nutmeg for garnish

1. Combine the water, apples, raisins, spices, and honey in a large soup pot or casserole and bring to a boil. Add the oats, cover, and reduce heat. Simmer for 45 minutes.

2. Stir in the lemon juice, brandy, and half the yogurt. Taste and adjust seasonings, adding more spices or honey if you wish.

3. Serve, garnishing each bowl with a dollop of yogurt, a thin slice of lemon, and a discreet sprinkle of nutmeg.

Delicate Lentil Soup

Serves 4

1 inch ball tamarind
¼ cup boiling water
1 onion, chopped
2 cloves garlic, minced or put through a press
1 tablespoon safflower oil
1 cup yellow lentils
4 cups water
2 cups chopped tomatoes (fresh or canned)
1 teaspoon molasses
1 tablespoon ground coriander
1 teaspoon ground cumin
¼ teaspoon ground black pepper
Cayenne to taste
Sea salt to taste
3 tablespoons chopped fresh coriander
Plain low-fat yogurt for garnish

1. Place the tamarind in a bowl and cover with ¼ cup boiling water. Let sit while you begin the soup.

2. Heat the safflower oil in a large, heavy-bottomed soup pot or casserole and add the onion and garlic. Sauté until the onion is tender and add the lentils, water, tomatoes, molasses, spices, and sea salt to taste. Bring to a boil. Reduce heat, cover, and simmer 30 minutes, or until the lentils are tender.

3. Meanwhile mash the tamarind pulp with the back of a spoon or with your fingers and strain the liquid through a fine strainer, making sure to squeeze out all the liquid. Add the juice to the lentils.

4. When the lentils are tender, purée in a blender. Then press through a fine strainer. Discard the pulp or save for another purpose, such as a bean spread. Return the liquid to the heat and heat through. Adjust seasonings and serve, garnishing each bowl with a dollop of plain, low-fat yogurt and a sprinkling of chopped fresh coriander.

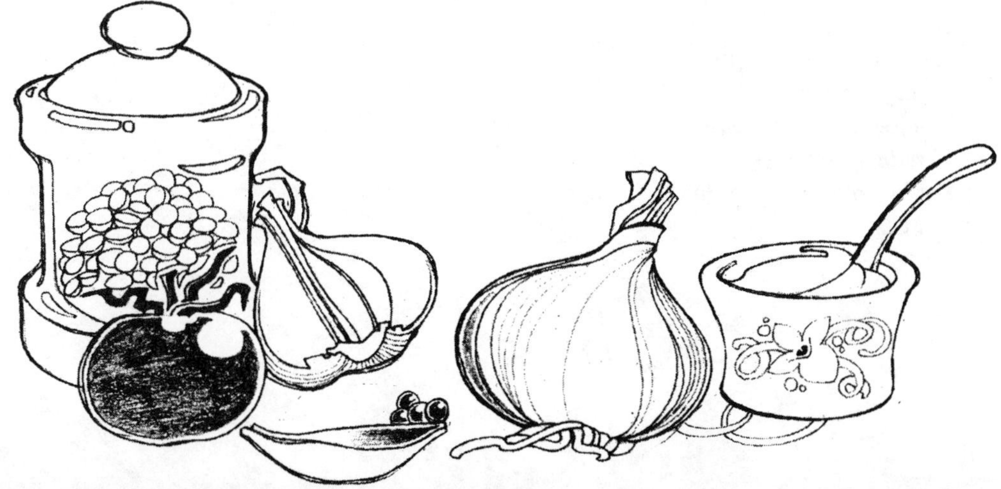

Cabbage-Apple Soup

Serves 4 to 6

1 tablespoon safflower oil
1 large onion, chopped
2 cloves garlic, minced or put through a press
1 teaspoon cinnamon
¼ teaspoon turmeric
¼ teaspoon ground cloves
1 to 2 teaspoons curry powder, to taste
1 pound red or green cabbage, shredded
6 cups water or ginger or regular vegetable stock (pages 54 and 55)
1 to 2 tablespoons soy sauce (optional)
Sea salt to taste
2 tart apples, cored and sliced
1 cup plain low-fat yogurt

For Garnish:
½ cup additional yogurt
½ additional apple, sliced thin and tossed with lemon juice
Freshly ground pepper to taste

1. Heat the safflower oil in a heavy-bottomed soup pot or Dutch oven and sauté the onion and garlic over medium heat until the onion begins to soften. Add the spices and sauté another 2 to 3 minutes, stirring. Add the cabbage and sauté another 5 minutes, stirring. Add the water or stock, the soy sauce, and salt to taste. Bring to a boil, reduce heat, cover, and simmer 30 minutes.

2. Add the apples and continue to simmer another 15 to 20 minutes. Taste and adjust seasoning, adding more salt or curry powder to taste. Remove from the heat, cool a minute, and stir in the yogurt and freshly ground pepper to taste. Serve, topping each bowl with a spoonful of yogurt and a few slices of apple.

Cabbage Soup Chinoise

Serves 4 to 6

5 cups ginger-vegetable stock (page 55) or vegetable bouillon
1 pound Chinese cabbage, shredded
6 green onions, thinly sliced
4 tablespoons soy sauce
2 tablespoons sherry
1 teaspoon grated fresh ginger
½ to 1 pound tofu, cut in cubes or slivers (optional)
1 tablespoon cornstarch dissolved in 2 tablespoons water
2 tablespoons sesame seeds and chopped fresh coriander for garnish

1. Place the stock in a large soup pot and bring to a simmer. Add the Chinese cabbage and green onions and simmer 5 minutes, or until the cabbage is cooked through but still has some texture.

2. Stir in the soy sauce, sherry, ginger, and tofu and heat through for 5 minutes. Stir in the cornstarch dissolved in the water and heat through, stirring, until the soup is thickened. Serve at once, garnishing each serving with sesame seeds and chopped fresh coriander.

Soupe au Coriandre

Serves 6 to 8

1 tablespoon olive oil
1 onion, chopped
2 cloves garlic, minced or put through a press
1 teaspoon ground cumin
1½ teaspoons paprika
1 32-ounce can tomatoes, chopped, with juice
4 cups water
4 tablespoons tomato paste
2 whole bunches coriander
Sea salt and freshly ground pepper to taste
½ cup vermicelli
Pinch of cayenne
Juice of 1 lime, or more, to taste

1. Keep the bunches of coriander gathered together so you can remove them after the soup simmers. Heat the olive oil in a large, heavy-bottomed soup pot or casserole and sauté the onion over medium-low heat until tender.

2. Add the garlic, cumin, and paprika, sauté a minute, and add the tomatoes and their juice, the water, the tomato paste, coriander, and sea salt and freshly ground pepper to taste. Bring to a simmer, cover, and simmer 30 minutes.

3. Remove the soup from the heat. Take out the coriander bunches and discard, and put the soup through a food mill. Return to the heat, bring back to a simmer, and add the vermicelli. Cook until al dente, adjust seasonings, and stir in the lime juice. Serve at once.

GUACAMOLE SOUP

Serves 6 to 8

1. Place all the ingredients except the yogurt and garnishes in a blender and blend until smooth. Transfer to a bowl and whisk in the yogurt (if you blend the yogurt with the other ingredients, the soup will be too thin). Adjust seasonings, adding more spices or salt to taste.

2. Cover and refrigerate for several hours before serving. Serve garnished with a dollop of yogurt and chopped fresh coriander.

3 cups tomato juice
1 tomato, peeled and quartered
1 small onion, quartered
1 jalapeño or serrano pepper, seeds removed
1 to 2 cloves garlic, to taste, peeled
3 large or 4 small ripe avocados, peeled and pitted
¼ cup lemon juice (juice of 1 large lemon)
1 teaspoon ground cumin
½ teaspoon chili powder (more to taste)
Sea salt to taste
2 cups plain low-fat yogurt
Additional yogurt and chopped fresh coriander for garnish

Potato-Cheese Soup with Cumin

Serves 6 to 8

1 tablespoon safflower oil, vegetable oil, or butter
4 leeks, white part only, cleaned and sliced thin
1 tablespoon cumin seeds, slightly crushed
2 pounds russet potatoes, unpeeled and diced
1 quart regular vegetable stock (page 54)
2 cups milk
Sea salt and freshly ground pepper to taste
6 ounces sharp cheddar or Gruyère cheese, grated
2 eggs, beaten

1. Heat the oil or butter over low heat in a large, heavy-bottomed soup pot or casserole and sauté the leeks for about 10 minutes, stirring often. Add the cumin seeds and sauté another minute or two, then add the potatoes and stock. Bring to a boil, reduce heat, cover, and simmer 30 minutes, or until the potatoes are tender.

2. With the back of your spoon, mash some of the potatoes against the side of the pot to thicken the soup a little. Stir in the milk, heat through, and add sea salt and freshly ground pepper to taste (remembering that the cheese will be salty).

3. Beat the eggs and stir in the cheese. Ladle some of the hot soup into the mixture, stir together, then stir the entire mixture into the soup. Heat through but do not boil, and serve.

Curried Cauliflower Soup

Serves 4 to 6

1 onion, chopped
1 clove garlic, minced or put through a press
1 tablespoon safflower oil
1 to 2 teaspoons curry powder, to taste
½ to 1 teaspoon ground cumin, to taste
¼ teaspoon turmeric
1 small head (about 1 ½ pounds) cauliflower, broken into florets
5 cups regular or ginger-vegetable stock (pages 54 and 55) or bouillon
1 small potato, peeled and diced
Sea salt to taste
1 cup plain, low-fat yogurt
1 teaspoon cornstarch
Freshly ground pepper to taste
Lemon juice to taste (optional)

1. Heat the oil in a soup pot and sauté the onion and garlic until the onion is tender. Add the curry powder, cumin, turmeric, and cauliflower and stir together for a minute or two. Add the stock or bouillon and the potato and bring to a boil. Cover, reduce heat, and simmer 30 minutes.

2. Purée in a blender or food processor in batches. Return to the pot and adjust seasonings, adding salt, pepper, curry powder or cumin to taste. Heat through.

3. Stir together the yogurt and cornstarch and whisk into the soup. Heat through and serve.

Hot and Sour Soup

Serves 6

- *6 dried Chinese mushrooms*
- *2 quarts ginger-vegetable stock (page 55)*
- *6 green onions, sliced, white and green parts separated*
- *½ pound tofu, slivered*
- *2 tablespoons dry sherry or Chinese rice wine*
- *¼ cup cider vinegar or Chinese rice wine vinegar (more to taste)*
- *2 to 3 tablespoons soy sauce, preferably tamari, or more to taste*
- *2 tablespoons cornstarch or arrowroot*
- *4 tablespoons water*
- *2 eggs, beaten*
- *1 large carrot, cut in 2-inch matchsticks*
- *1 stalk celery or bok choy, cut in 2-inch matchsticks*
- *½ cup cucumber, cut in matchsticks*
- *¼ to ½ teaspoon freshly ground black pepper, to taste*
- *2 tablespoons chopped fresh coriander*

1. Before you begin cutting the vegetables, place the mushrooms in a small bowl. Bring 2 cups of the stock to a boil and pour over the mushrooms. Let stand for 15 minutes while you prepare the remaining ingredients.

2. Place the remaining ginger-vegetable stock in a large soup pot or casserole. Drain the mushrooms and retain the soaking liquid. Strain this through a cheesecloth or coffee filter and add it to the stock. Cut the mushrooms in slivers and add them to the stock, along with the white part of the green onions. Simmer 5 minutes and add the tofu. Simmer 5 more minutes and stir in the sherry, vinegar, and tamari soy sauce.

3. Dissolve the cornstarch or arrowroot in the water. Stir this into the soup, bring to a gentle boil, and cook, stirring, until the soup thickens, about 3 minutes.

4. Drizzle the beaten eggs into the simmering soup, stirring with a fork or chopstick so that the eggs form shreds. Remove the soup from the heat, stir in the pepper, taste, and adjust vinegar, soy sauce, and pepper.

5. Distribute carrots, bok choy or celery, cucumber, and green onion tops among the bowls and ladle in the soup. Sprinkle a little fresh coriander on each bowlful and serve at once, passing additional pepper and vinegar so people can adjust the hot and sour to their tastes.

Sopa de Tortilla

Serves 6 to 8

3 chilies pasillas
2 tablespoons safflower oil
½ onion, minced
4 cloves garlic, minced or put through a press
1 tablespoon olive oil
6 cups regular vegetable stock (page 54)
2 tomatoes, peeled, seeded, and puréed
4 tablespoons tomato paste
Pinch of cayenne
Additional safflower or vegetable oil
12 stale corn tortillas, cut in strips
3 tablespoons chopped fresh coriander, plus more for garnish
Sea salt and freshly ground pepper to taste
2 ounces Gruyère cheese, grated
2 eggs, beaten

1. Heat 2 tablespoons safflower oil in a heavy-bottomed frying pan and fry the chilies pasillas until crisp. Remove from the heat and, when cool enough to handle, crumble, discard seeds, and set aside.

2. Heat the olive oil in a heavy-bottomed soup pot or casserole and add the onion and garlic. Cook over medium heat until the onion is tender. Add the puréed tomato and the tomato paste. Cook over low heat for 8 to 10 minutes, and add the vegetable stock. Stir together well, add the cayenne, and bring to a simmer. Cover and simmer over low heat for 30 minutes.

3. Meanwhile, heat ¼ inch of safflower oil in a frying pan and sauté the tortilla strips in batches (don't crowd the pan), until just crisp. Drain on paper towels.

4. Shortly before serving the soup, stir in the fried tortilla strips. Simmer for a minute or two, then add the coriander and sea salt and freshly ground pepper to taste.

5. Put some crumbled fried chilies pasillas in each bowl. Bring the soup to a boil and stir in the eggs. They should cook at once. Immediately spoon the soup into the bowls, top with cheese and a little more coriander if you wish, and serve.

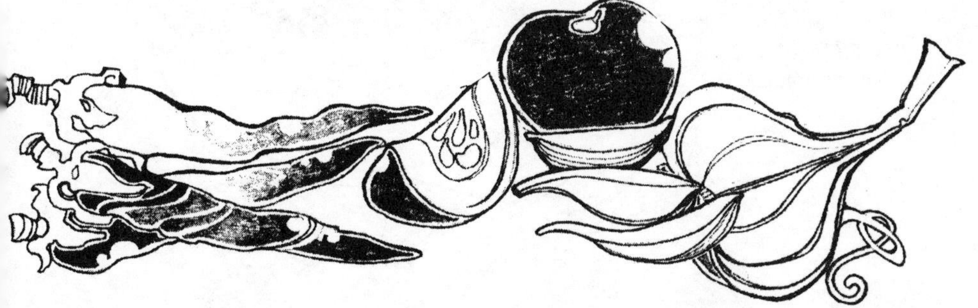

Indian Split Pea Soup

The flavor of this subtle, beautifully colored soup is greatly enhanced by the lemon juice which you sprinkle on each bowl just before serving.

Serves 4

1 tablespoon black peppercorns
12 cloves
1 bay leaf, crushed
1 tablespoon safflower or vegetable oil, or butter
1 small onion, minced
1 teaspoon mustard seeds
½ pound split peas, washed and picked over
½ teaspoon turmeric
5 cups plain or ginger-vegetable stock (pages 54 and 55) or water
Sea salt and freshly ground pepper to taste
2 tablespoons milk or cream (optional)
Juice of ½ lemon
1 lemon, cut in wedges, for garnish
Croûtons, for garnish
Plain low-fat yogurt for garnish (optional)

1. Tie the black peppercorns, the cloves, and the bay leaves in cheesecloth and set aside.

2. Heat the oil in a heavy-bottomed soup pot or casserole and sauté the onion with the mustard seeds over medium heat until the onion is tender. Add the split peas, the turmeric, the stock or water, salt to taste, and the spices in their cheesecloth bag. Bring to a boil, reduce heat, and simmer 45 minutes to an hour, or until the peas are tender.

3. Remove the cheesecloth bag from the soup and squeeze out all the liquid. Purée the soup in a blender or through a food mill. Return to the pot and heat through.

4. Correct seasonings, adding salt and freshly group pepper to taste, and stir in the optional milk or cream. Serve, sprinkling fresh lemon juice over each bowl and garnishing with lemon wedges, croûtons, and optional plain low-fat yogurt.

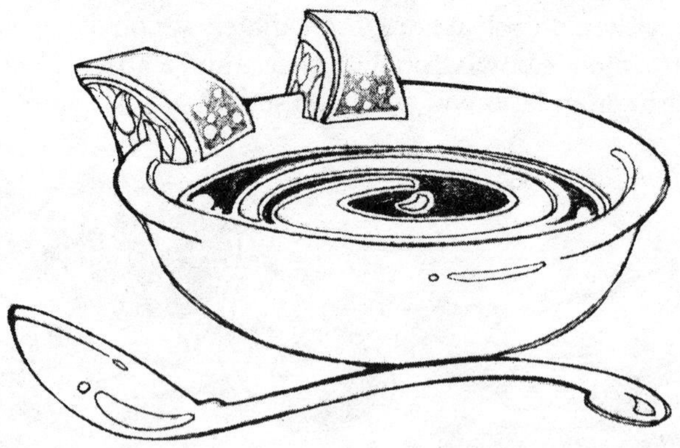

HUMMUS SOUP

Since I love all the flavors of hummus, the spread made with garbanzos, lemon, garlic, olive oil, and tahini, I decided to see if they would translate into a soup. They did. This tastes best if served the day after it's made.

Serves 6

½ pound garbanzos, washed, picked over and soaked overnight
6 cups water
½ teaspoon turmeric
1 teaspoon ground cumin
½ teaspoon ground coriander
Pinch of saffron
1 teaspoon, or more to taste, sea salt
2 large cloves garlic (more to taste), peeled
Juice of 2 lemons (¼ to ⅔ cup lemon juice, to taste)
5 to 6 tablespoons sesame tahini (to taste)
1 cup plain low-fat yogurt, plus additional for garnish
Additional lemon wedges for garnish

1. Soak the garbanzos overnight in three times their volume of water. Drain them and combine with the water, turmeric, cumin, and coriander in a large, heavy-bottomed soup pot. Bring to a boil and add the saffron. Cover, reduce heat, and simmer 1 hour. Add the sea salt and continue to simmer another hour, or until the beans are tender.

2. Blend the soup to a smooth purée in a blender or food processor, along with the garlic, lemon juice, and sesame tahini. Pour back into the pot and whisk in the yogurt. Thin out, if you wish, with water or additional yogurt. Taste and adjust seasonings. Heat through and serve, topping each bowl with a spoonful of yogurt and a sprinkling of lemon juice.

Tomato-Lentil Rasam

A "rasam" is a highly seasoned South Indian broth made from the liquid which rises to the top when lentils, tomatoes, and spices are cooked. This recipe is based on Julie Sahni's in Classic Indian Cooking. *The "Delicate Lentil Soup" on page 61 is a thicker, less spicy version of this rasam.*

Serves 4 to 6

1 cup yellow lentils (toovar dal), washed and picked over
1 teaspoon turmeric
1 pound chopped tomatoes, fresh or canned
6 cloves garlic, peeled
A 1-inch ball of tamarind pulp (substitute juice of 1 lemon if you can't find tamarind)
1 teaspoon ground cumin
¼ teaspoon black pepper
⅛ to ¼ teaspoon cayenne pepper (to taste)
1 tablespoon ground coriander
1 teaspoon honey or molasses
Sea salt to taste
1 tablespoon safflower or vegetable oil
1 teaspoon black mustard seeds
⅛ teaspoon ground asafetida (optional)

1. Combine the lentils and 4 cups of water in a large saucepan and bring to a boil. Cover, reduce heat, and simmer for about 35 minutes, or until the lentils are tender. Stir occasionally to prevent sticking.

2. Meanwhile place the tamarind pulp in a bowl and pour on ¼ cup boiling water. Let sit for 15 minutes. Strain the liquid into a bowl through a fine strainer, mashing the tamarind pulp against the sides of the strainer in order to extrude the maximum amount of juice.

3. While the lentils are simmering and the tamarind soaking, purée the tomatoes and garlic with ½ cup cold water and the turmeric, cumin, coriander, black pepper, and cayenne in a blender or food processor. Set aside.

4. When the lentils are tender, purée in a blender or food processor or through a food mill, and return to the pot. Blend in 3 cups hot water with a whisk, mix thoroughly, and allow the mixture to sit, undisturbed, for 15 minutes. A broth will accumulate at the top, and this is the broth you want. Pour off the broth and add enough water to measure 4½ cups. Transfer the lentil purée that remains to a bowl and save for another purpose. Return the broth to the pot and stir in the blended tomatoes and spices, the molasses or honey, the

tamarind juice, and sea salt to taste. Bring to a boil, reduce heat, and simmer, partially covered, over low heat for 15 minutes. Remove from the heat.

2 to 3 tablespoons chopped fresh coriander

5. Heat the oil over high heat in a small frying pan, and when it is very hot, carefully add the mustard seeds. Keep a lid handy to protect yourself from spluttering oil. As soon as the seeds stop sputtering and turn gray—which will only take a few seconds—transfer the contents of the pan to the soup, cover the soup, and let sit another 15 minutes.

6. To serve the soup, reheat to a simmer while stirring, adjust salt and cayenne, stir in the coriander, and serve.

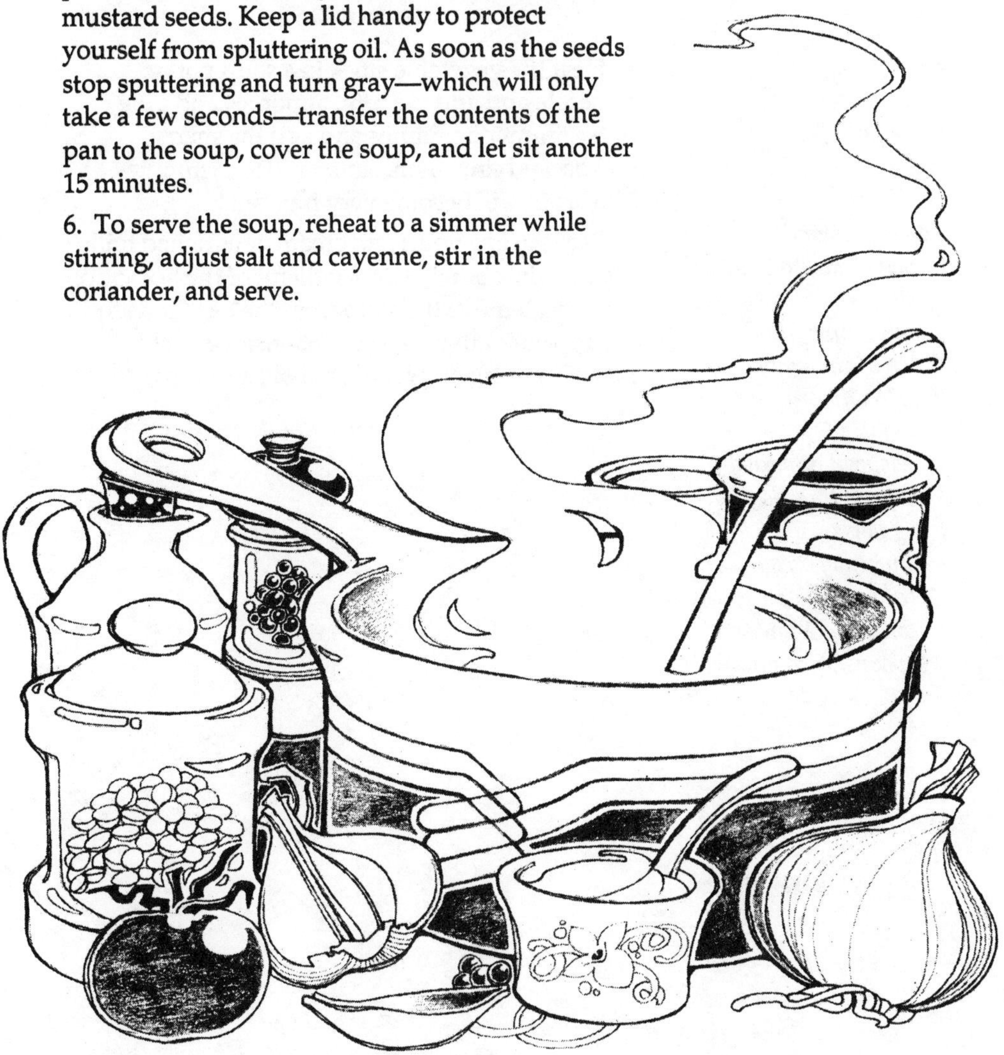

Rich Saffron Soup

This soup has an unbelievably beautiful color. The almonds and pine nuts give it a great texture, but if you want a lighter soup you may omit them.

Serves 6 to 8

2 quarts regular vegetable stock (page 54)
½ pound tofu, cut in slivers
1 ounce almonds, blanched and cut in slivers
½ ounce pine nuts
Pinch of cinnamon
¼ to ½ cup dry sherry, to taste
½ teaspoon imported saffron threads
2 egg yolks
½cup heavy cream (or use milk enriched with 1 to 2 tablespoons dried milk)

1. Heat the vegetable stock in a soup pot or casserole and add the tofu, almonds, and pine nuts. Simmer 5 minutes and add the sherry, saffron, and cinnamon. Simmer 10 to 15 minutes. The broth will become very fragrant.

2. Beat the egg yolks and cream or enriched milk together in a bowl. Add a ladleful of the hot soup, stirring. Remove the soup from the heat and stir in the egg yolk mixture. Serve at once, or heat through, being careful not to boil, and serve.

Velvet Corn Soup with Green Chili

Serves 4

1. Combine the corn kernels, milk, and honey in a heavy-bottomed saucepan and simmer over low heat for 15 minutes, stirring occasionally. Remove from the heat and purée in a blender or food processor. Mixture will be like thick creamed corn.

2. Heat the oil in a heavy-bottomed saucepan or casserole and add the green onions, chili peppers, and ginger. Sauté, stirring for 1 minute, and add the vegetable stock, corn purée, sherry, optional sesame oil, and pepper. Mix together well. Bring to a simmer and simmer 5 minutes.

3. Dissolve the cornstarch in the water and stir into the soup. Cook, stirring, until the soup thickens, about 3 minutes. Remove from the heat and adjust seasonings.

4. Beat the egg whites until frothy and slowly drizzle them into the soup while you stir with a fork or wooden spoon so they cook in delicate threads. Ladle into warm bowls, garnish with chopped fresh coriander, and serve at once.

3 cups corn kernels, fresh or thawed frozen
1½ cups milk (whole or low-fat)
1 tablespoon mild-flavored honey
1 tablespoon safflower, peanut, or vegetable oil
3 green onions with tops, sliced on the diagonal
1 to 2 hot green chili peppers, to taste, seeded and thinly sliced
1 teaspoon minced fresh ginger
3 cups regular or ginger-vegetable stock (pages 54 and 55)
2 tablespoons good quality sherry or Chinese rice wine
Sea salt to taste
½ teaspoon sesame oil (optional)
A generous amount of freshly ground white or black pepper
1 tablespoon cornstarch
2 tablespoons water
2 egg whites, lightly beaten
3 tablespoons chopped fresh coriander

Sweet and Sour Cabbage Soup

This is a vegetarian version of the enticing "Jewish Sweet and Sour Soup" in Richard Sax's Cooking Great Meals Every Day *(Random House, New York, 1982).*

Serves 4 to 6

2 tablespoons safflower or vegetable oil
2 medium onions, sliced
1 medium-sized cabbage, cored and cut in strips
½ cup golden raisins
Juice of 2 small or medium lemons (about ⅓ cup), more to taste
2 tablespoons mild-tasting honey
2 cloves garlic, minced or put through a press
Sea salt to taste
2 teaspoons Hungarian paprika
¼ teaspoon ground cloves
1 2-pound can tomatoes, with their liquid
4 cups water or regular vegetable stock (page 54)
2 tablespoons soy sauce
2 slices dark pumpernickel bread, diced
Freshly ground black pepper to taste
Pinch of cayenne (optional)
Plain low-fat yogurt for garnish

1. Heat the oil over medium-low heat in a large, heavy-bottomed soup pot or casserole and add the onions. Sauté, stirring often, until the onions are soft, about 10 minutes.

2. Meanwhile prepare the cabbage and combine the raisins, lemon juice, and honey in a small bowl.

3. Add the garlic, cabbage, and salt to the pot with the sautéed onions, stir together well, cover, and sauté, stirring from time to time, for about 4 minutes.

4. Add the paprika, cloves, and tomatoes, and stir together well. Add the water or vegetable stock, soy sauce, more salt to taste, the raisin/lemon juice mixture, and the bread, and bring to a simmer. Cover and simmer for 45 minutes to an hour, stirring from time to time.

5. Taste and adjust seasonings, adding freshly group pepper to taste and a pinch of cayenne if you wish. Serve, garnishing each bowl with plain low-fat yogurt.

PIQUANT CHICK PEA SOUP

Serves 6

1 pound garbanzos, picked over, washed and soaked overnight
1 large onion, chopped
3 large cloves garlic (more to taste), minced or put through a press
1 tablespoon olive oil
5 cups water
1 pound tomatoes, fresh or canned, chopped
4 tablespoons tomato paste
1 rind of Parmesan cheese
1 bay leaf
1 small, dried, hot red pepper, such as cayenne
½ teaspoon thyme
½ teaspoon oregano
Sea salt and freshly ground pepper to taste
Chopped fresh parsley for garnish

1. Combine the soaked garbanzos with 6 cups water, bring to a boil, reduce heat, and simmer, covered, for 1 hour. Drain and set aside.

2. Heat the olive oil in a heavy-bottomed soup pot and sauté the onion and one clove of the garlic until the onion is tender. Add the garbanzos, 5 cups water, tomatoes, tomato paste, Parmesan cheese, bay leaf, and hot red pepper, and bring to a boil. Reduce heat, cover, and simmer 1 to 2 hours, or until the beans are tender. Add the thyme, oregano, sea salt and pepper to taste, cayenne, and more garlic if you wish, and continue to simmer another 20 minutes. Serve garnished with chopped fresh parsley.

Almond Soup

This soup is from my cookbook The Vegetarian Feast. *Each spice is distinctive, yet the overall flavor of the soup is subtle. It is a rich soup with great texture.*

Serves 4 to 6

1 quart regular or ginger-vegetable stock (pages 54 and 55)
2 cups whole almonds, blanched
1 medium onion, chopped
1 tablespoon butter or safflower oil
Grated rind of 1 to 2 lemons, to taste
½ teaspoon ground cardamom
½ teaspoon caraway seeds
Sea salt and freshly ground pepper to taste
2 cups milk
1 teaspoon lemon juice
1 cup cooked, long-grain brown rice
½ cup currants
Freshly grated nutmeg to taste

1. Using enough stock to cover, purée the blanched almonds, a cup at a time, in a blender until coarsely ground. They should retain some texture but should be finer than chopped almonds.

2. Heat the butter or oil in a heavy-bottomed soup pot or casserole and sauté the onion until tender. Add the almonds, remaining stock, grated lemon peel, cardamom, caraway seeds, sea salt, and pepper. Cover and simmer gently for 30 minutes, stirring occasionally.

3. Carefully add the milk and lemon juice, and correct the seasonings. Add the rice and currants and simmer very gently for another 10 minutes. Grate some nutmeg over the top and serve, or chill and serve cold, grating additional nutmeg over each serving.

Peach Soup

This recipe is also in my Herb and Honey Cookery. *It is such a good example of a summer soup that makes the most of sweet spices that I couldn't resist including it in this collection.*

Serves 6 to 8

3 pounds fresh, ripe peaches
3 to 4 tablespoons mild-flavored honey, to taste
1 cup orange juice
3 tablespoons peach brandy or marsala
3 tablespoons lemon or lime juice (more to taste)
¾ teaspoon cinnamon
½ teaspoon freshly grated nutmeg
¼ teaspoon ground ginger
½ teaspoon ground cardamom
½ to 1 teaspoon vanilla, to taste
5 cups buttermilk
½ cup slivered almonds, for garnish

1. Blanch the peaches in boiling water, refresh immediately in cold water, and remove the skins. Set aside six peaches.

2. Pit the remaining peaches and combine with the honey, orange juice, brandy or marsala, lemon or lime juice, spices, and vanilla. Purée in a blender or food processor. Transfer to a large bowl and stir in the buttermilk.

3. Slice the peaches that were set aside and add to the soup. Cover and chill several hours.

4. Adjust seasonings and serve, garnishing each bowl with slivered almonds.

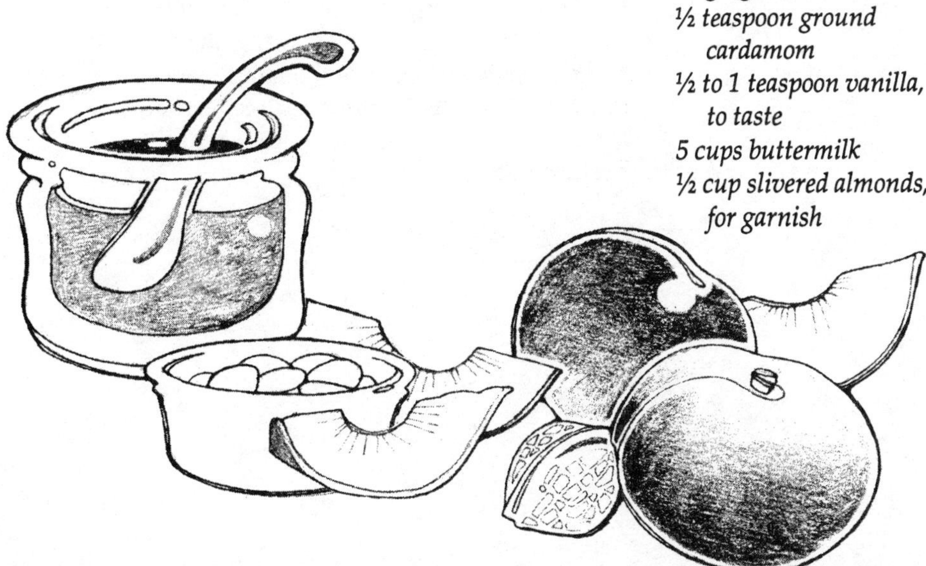

3
VEGETABLES

Cauliflower à la Saffron

Serves 4

1 large head cauliflower, broken into florets (cut the florets into halves or quarters if very large)
3 cups water
¼ teaspoon saffron
¼ teaspoon sea salt (more to taste)
2 tablespoons butter
2 tablespoons whole wheat pastry flour

1. Bring 1 cup of the water to a boil. Place the saffron in a small bowl and pour on the boiling water. Let steep for 10 to 15 minutes.

2. Bring the remaining water to a boil in a saucepan. Add the saffron water, sea salt, and cauliflower. Cover and cook 10 minutes. Drain and retain the cooking liquid, which you will use for a sauce.

3. In a heavy-bottomed saucepan melt the butter over medium heat. Add the flour and stir together well with a wooden spoon. Cook, stirring, for a minute or two. Now whisk in the liquid from the cauliflower. Bring to a boil, stirring all the while, and reduce heat. Stir until the sauce reaches the desired thickness. Add more salt to taste and freshly ground pepper, toss with the cauliflower, heat through, and serve.

SPICY EGGPLANT AND SNOW PEAS WITH MISO

Serves 6

½ pound snow peas, trimmed
4 tablespoons hatcho miso
3 tablespoons water
1 tablespoon mild-flavored honey
1 teaspoon sesame oil
1 medium-sized egg-plant, peeled and diced small
2 tablespoons safflower or vegetable oil
2 cloves garlic, minced or put through a press
2 teaspoons minced or grated fresh ginger
8 green onions, both white part and green, sliced
½ teaspoon hot red pepper flakes, or 1 small dried red pepper, crumbled, seeds removed

1. Steam the peas for 5 to 10 minutes, to taste. Refresh under cold water and set aside.

2. In a small bowl mix together the miso, water, honey, and sesame oil. Set aside.

3. Heat the oil in a wok or a large, heavy-bottomed frying pan and add the eggplant. Sauté for 5 minutes, stirring. Add the garlic and ginger and sauté another 10 minutes, stirring. Add the miso mixture and continue to stir-fry for another 3 to 5 minutes, then add the onions and pepper flakes or crumbled pepper and cook, stirring, until the onions and eggplant are tender. If necessary, add a little more oil or 2 to 3 tablespoons water. Add the snow peas, toss together well, heat through, and serve over hot, cooked grains.

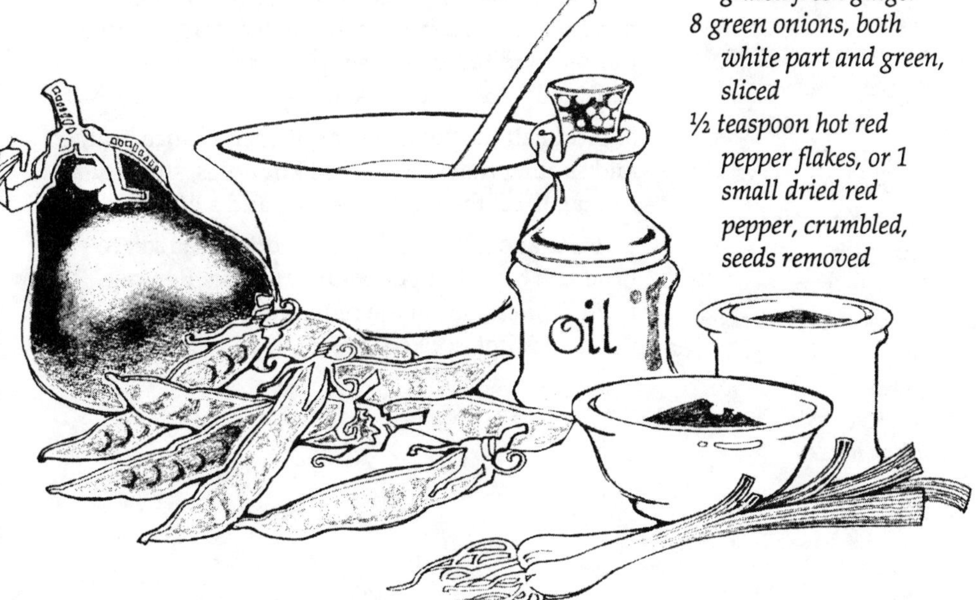

EGGPLANT AND RED PEPPERS WITH FRAGRANT SPICES

The eggplant has an almost puréed consistency in this marvelously perfumed dish. The strips of sweet red pepper lend a beautiful contrast of colors.

3 pounds eggplant, cut in half lengthwise
1 tablespoon flour
2 to 3 tablespoons safflower or vegetable oil, as needed
1 large onion, sliced thin
1 sweet red pepper, seeded and cut in lengthwise strips
2 tablespoons minced fresh ginger
4 cloves garlic, minced or put through a press
1½ teaspoons ground cumin
1½ teaspoons ground mace or nutmeg
¾ teaspoon ground cinnamon
1 teaspoon Mughal garam masala (see page 26)
1 teaspoon paprika
Cayenne pepper to taste
2 cups plain low-fat yogurt
Sea salt to taste
Milk as needed

1. Preheat the oven to 450°F. Oil a baking sheet. Score the halved eggplants once or twice, down to the skin but not through it. Place cut side down on the baking sheets and bake 15 minutes, or until the skins begin to shrivel. Meanwhile, prepare remaining ingredients. Remove the eggplants from the oven and allow to cool. When cool enough to handle, scoop out from the skin, cut in dice, and toss in a bowl with 1 tablespoon flour.

2. Heat the oil over medium heat in a large, wide, preferably nonstick frying pan and add the onion. Sauté until golden, about 5 to 10 minutes, and add the red pepper, garlic, and ginger. Cook, stirring, for about 2 minutes, and stir in the spices. Cook for about 30 seconds, and add the eggplant and more oil (about a tablespoon) if necessary. Turn up the heat and brown the eggplant, stirring constantly, for about 5 minutes.

3. Add half the yogurt, stir together, reduce heat, and simmer the mixture for 15 minutes, stirring frequently. If the mixture sticks, add a little milk.

4. Taste and adjust the spices, adding sea salt to taste and more hot pepper if you wish. Remove from the heat, stir in the remaining yogurt, and serve with hot, cooked grains.

Nutty Eggplant and Potato Curry

Serves 6 to 8

1½ pounds eggplant, cut in half lengthwise
2 tablespoons butter, safflower oil, or vegetable oil
1 medium-sized onion, sliced
½ pound potatoes, diced
1 clove garlic, minced or put through a press
1 teaspoon minced fresh ginger, or ¼ teaspoon dried
1 tablespoon curry powder
¼ cup peanuts, almonds, or sunflower seeds
½ cup raisins
1 cup buttermilk or plain yogurt
Sea salt and freshly ground pepper to taste
2 tablespoons chopped fresh coriander

1. Preheat the oven to 450°F. Oil a baking sheet. Score the eggplant halves down the middle, to the skin but not through it. Place cut side down on the baking sheets, pop in the preheated oven, and bake 10 to 15 minutes, or until the skins begin to shrivel. Remove from the heat and allow to cool until you can handle them, then dice.

2. Meanwhile steam the potatoes until crisp-tender, 10 to 15 minutes.

3. Heat the butter or oil in a heavy-bottomed frying pan or wok and add the onion, garlic, and ginger. Sauté over medium-low heat for a minute or two, then add the curry powder. Sauté gently for about 15 minutes, stirring.

4. Add the steamed potato and eggplant, raisins, nuts, and more oil or butter if necessary, and sauté, stirring, for another 10 minutes. Add sea salt and freshly ground pepper to taste, remove from the heat, cool a moment, and stir in the yogurt or buttermilk and the chopped, fresh coriander. Serve over hot, cooked grains.

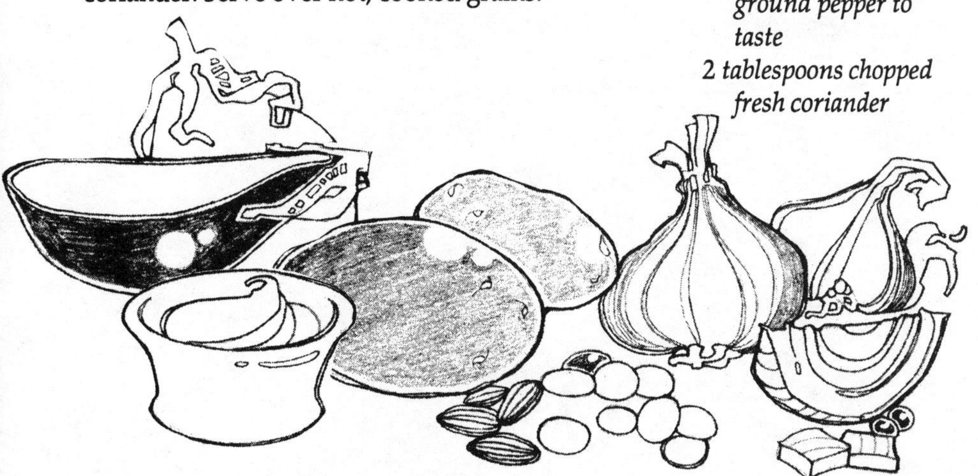

Spicy Potatoes in Yogurt Gravy

Serves 8

2 pounds new or red waxy potatoes, cut in large chunks
2 tablespoons safflower or light vegetable oil
2 onions, finely chopped
1 tablespoon minced fresh ginger root
2 teaspoons ground cumin
2 teaspoons ground coriander
1 teaspoon turmeric
¼ teaspoon cayenne
1 teaspoon Mughal garam masala (page 26)
1 pound chopped or puréed tomatoes, fresh or canned
1½ cups plain low-fat yogurt
Sea salt to taste

1. Steam the potatoes until crisp-tender, about 10 minutes. Drain and set aside.

2. Have the spices measured out and ready, right next to the stove. Heat the oil in a large, heavy-bottomed casserole or lidded frying pan and add the onions. Stir-fry, stirring constantly, for 10 minutes over medium-low heat or until they begin to turn light brown. Add the ginger and fry for an additional ½ minute (add more oil if necessary), then add all the spices and stir together for another 30 seconds. Add the potatoes, tomatoes, half the yogurt, and salt to taste, and bring to a boil. Reduce heat and simmer gently, covered, for about 30 minutes, or until the potatoes are tender. Stir from time to time to prevent sticking.

3. Remove from the heat, let sit a minute, and stir in the remaining yogurt. Adjust salt and serve.

Note: This is best made a few hours or a day before and reheated gently.

Spicy Potatoes in Gravy

This dish is somewhere between a thick soup and a vegetable dish. I love the warming flavors. I serve it as a vegetable course, but in bowls. You could also serve it over rice.

Serves 4

1½ pounds new or red waxy potatoes, diced
3 tablespoons safflower or light vegetable oil
1 teaspoon black mustard seeds
2 teaspoons yellow split peas (channa dal, optional)
2 tablespoons minced fresh ginger
1 to 2 green chilies, seeded and sliced, or ¼ teaspoon cayenne (optional)
1 tablespoon ground coriander
1 teaspoon turmeric
½ teaspoon paprika
2 onions, chopped
Sea salt to taste
4 tablespoons chopped fresh coriander
Juice of 1 lemon, or more, to taste

1. Steam the potatoes until tender, about 20 minutes. Drain and refresh under cold water, and set aside.

2. Have the spices measured out and ready, right next to the stove.

3. Heat the oil over medium heat in a large, heavy-bottomed saucepan or deep, lidded frying pan. Add the mustard seeds and cook until they begin to turn gray and the sputtering begins to subside. Add the optional split peas and fry until light brown, about ½ to 1 minute, stirring constantly. Add the ginger and chilies, cook for 1 minute, and add the ground coriander, turmeric, and paprika. Stir together and add the onions. Sauté, stirring, for 5 minutes or until mixture begins to brown. Add potatoes and fry 5 minutes, adding more oil if necessary.

4. Add 4 cups hot water and sea salt to taste, and bring to a simmer. Simmer, covered, over low heat for 15 minutes, or until the potatoes are tender.

5. Remove 1½ cups of the mixture and purée in a blender or food processor, or put through a food mill. Return to the pot and mix together well. Adjust salt. Heat through, stirring (a layer may stick to the bottom of the pot, but don't let this worry you).

6. Stir in the lemon juice and coriander and serve at once, in bowls.

Vegetable Fritters

These are a spicy version of tempura. You can use just one vegetable such as onions for onion fritters, or cauliflower, or a combination such as broccoli, zucchini, carrots, onions, and cauliflower.

Serves 6 to 10

For the Batter:

¾ cup whole wheat pastry or unbleached white flour (don't use a coarse flour or the batter will be too heavy)
¼ cup garbanzo flour (use 1 cup whole wheat pastry or unbleached white in all if garbanzo flour is unavailable)
2 teaspoons ground or crushed coriander seeds
Pinch of cayenne
¼ teaspoon ground cumin
¾ teaspoon sea salt
2 tablespoons safflower, sesame, or vegetable oil
2 eggs, separated
1 cup water

Oil for deep-frying

1. First make the batter. Combine the flours, salt, spices, oil, egg yolks, and water. Stir together but don't beat. Let stand for 20 minutes. Then beat the egg whites until fluffy and fold them into the batter.

2. Blanch the broccoli and cauliflower and drain well.

3. Toss the vegetables in a bowl with the additional flour. If the carrots are grated, take them up in clumps and dip them in the flour. You will then dip them in the batter to deep-fry them in clumps.

4. Heat the oil in a wok or deep-fryer to 370°F. When it is hot, dip the vegetables into the batter, roll them around to coat evenly, and deep-fry a few at a time. They should float to the top and turn a golden brown very quickly. Remove them from the oil with a slotted spoon, allowing excess oil to drip back into the pan, and drain on paper towels. Make sure to let the oil come back up to 370°F. between batches.

5. Keep the fritters warm in a low oven. Serve when all are done with soy sauce.

Note: This can be held for an hour or so. Just before serving, heat the oil again, drop in or a few seconds to crisp, drain, and serve.

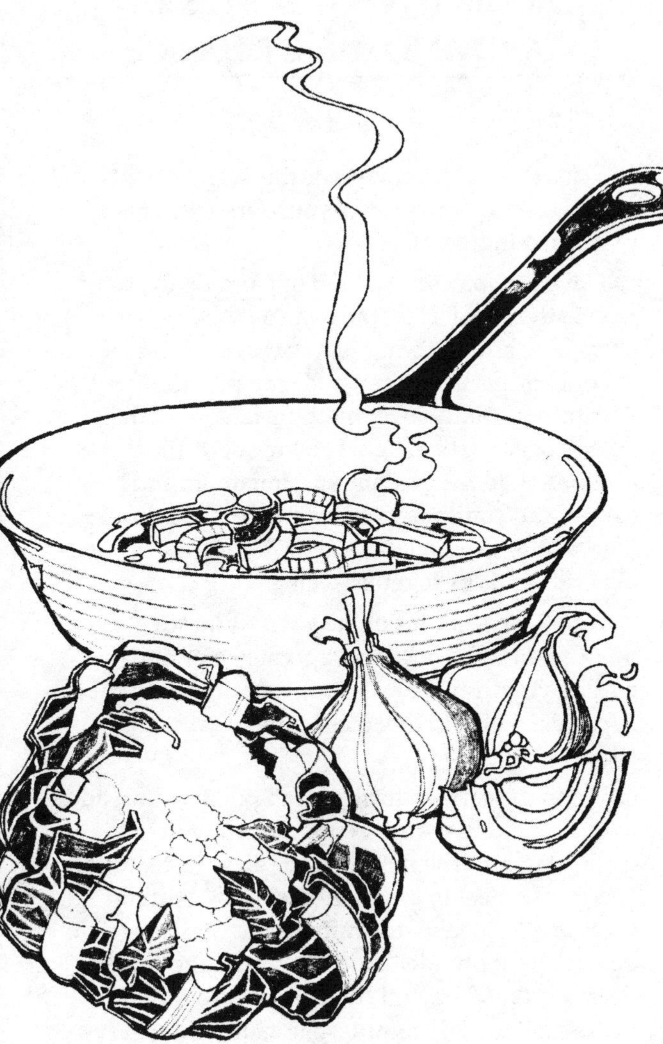

For Mixed Vegetable Fritters:

½ head broccoli, broken into florets

½ small head cauliflower, broken into florets

1 onion, sliced in rings

1 to 2 zucchini, sliced

1 to 2 carrots, sliced or grated

½ cup unbleached white flour

For Onion Fritters:

2 pounds onions, sliced in rings

½ cup unbleached white flour

For Cauliflower Fritters:

1 large head cauliflower, broken into florets

½ cup unbleached white flour

Braised Vegetables in Cardamom Nut Sauce

Serves 4 to 6

½ pound potatoes, peeled and diced
½ pound turnips, peeled and diced
1 carrot, peeled and diced
2 tablespoons safflower or light vegetable oil
2 medium-sized onions, finely chopped
2 large cloves garlic, minced
1 tablespoon minced fresh ginger
1 green chili, seeded and minced
12 green or 9 white cardamom pods
1 stick cinnamon, 3 inches long
24 whole cloves
5 tablespoons ground, blanched almonds
1 cup plain low-fat yogurt
1 cup shelled fresh green or frozen peas, defrosted
Salt to taste
¼ cup heavy cream

1. Place the diced potatoes, turnips, and carrots in a bowl of cold water while you work with the remaining ingredients.

2. Have the spices measured out and ready, right next to the stove. Heat the oil in a large, heavy-bottomed, lidded frying pan or casserole and add the onions, garlic, ginger, and chili pepper. Sauté, stirring constantly, over medium heat until the onions begin to turn light brown, about 10 minutes. Add the cardamom, cinnamon, and cloves, and continue to stir-fry another 5 minutes (add a little more oil if necessary). Add the ground almonds and stir together well.

3. Add 2 tablespoons of the yogurt and stir-fry the mixture until the yogurt evaporates. Continue adding yogurt in 2-tablespoon amounts until the cup is used up, stirring constantly to avoid sticking.

4. Drain the carrots, turnips, and potatoes and add to the pot along with 1½ cups hot water. If using fresh peas, add them now. Add salt to taste, cover, and reduce heat to medium-low. Cook, stirring occasionally, for about 30 minutes, or until the vegetables are tender. Add the cream and frozen peas, stir together, and cook uncovered for 10 minutes. If after 10 minutes the sauce is not very thick, increase heat to medium and simmer until it reaches the desired con-sistency. If it is too thick, thin out with a little hot water or milk. Correct salt and serve over hot cooked grains.

Note: This tastes best if prepared a day ahead and will keep in the refrigerator for up to 4 days.

TZIMMES

Tzimmes (pronounced "tsimmis") is a traditional Jewish sweet potato casserole. It appears at Jewish holiday dinners but needn't be reserved for these days.

Serves 6

3 large sweet potatoes, well scrubbed
1 cup plain low-fat yogurt
3 tablespoons butter
½ pound carrots, peeled and grated
½ pound tart apples, peeled, cored, and grated
2 tablespoons mild-flavored honey
⅔ cup raisins
½ cup chopped walnuts or pecans
½ teaspoon cinnamon
¼ teaspoon ground cloves
¼ teaspoon ground nutmeg
¼ teaspoon sea salt

1. Preheat the oven to 425°F. Bake the potatoes in their skins until thoroughly tender, about 45 minutes. Remove from the oven and reduce heat to 350°F.
2. Scoop out the potato from the peel, discard the peels, and purée the potatoes in a food pro-cessor fitted with the steel blade, or through a food mill. Mix in the yogurt and 1 tablespoon of butter. Set aside.
3. Heat the remaining butter in a heavy-bottomed casserole or frying pan and add the carrots. Sauté, stirring, for about 5 minutes, then stir in the apples and sauté another 5 minutes. Remove from the heat and add the honey, raisins, nuts, spices, and sea salt. Stir in the sweet potato purée and mix everything together well.
4. Transfer to an oiled or buttered baking dish or casserole, cover with foil or a lid, and bake in the preheated oven for 20 to 30 minutes. Serve hot.

Celery au Cumin

Serves 4

1 pound celery, washed and sliced
Juice of 2 lemons
¼ cup olive oil
¾ teaspoon ground cumin
Pinch of sea salt
Freshly ground pepper, to taste
Minced fresh parsley, for garnish

1. Heat the lemon juice and olive oil in a heavy-bottomed lidded casserole. Add the remaining ingredients, stir together well, cover, and simmer over low heat for 20 to 30 minutes.

2. Remove from the heat, transfer to a bowl, and chill several hours. Sprinkle with parsley and serve.

Steamed Peas with Mild Yogurt Sauce

Serves 4

1½ pounds fresh peas, shelled
1 cup plain, low-fat yogurt
1 teaspoon ground cumin
½ teaspoon ground coriander
Sea salt to taste
2 teaspoons lemon juice

1. Steam the peas until tender, about 10 to 15 minutes.

2. Meanwhile, mix together the yogurt, spices, and sea salt to taste. Stir in the lemon juice.

3. When the peas are done, drain and toss at once with the sauce. Serve.

Peas with Ginger, Spices, and Fresh Coriander

Serves 6

2½ pounds fresh peas, shelled
2 tablespoons safflower or peanut oil
¼ teaspoon whole black mustard seeds
5 whole fenugreek seeds
1 piece fresh ginger, about 2 inches long, peeled and finely minced or grated
¼ teaspoon ground turmeric
1 teaspoon ground coriander
1 teaspoon ground cumin
1 teaspoon garam masala (see page 27)
Sea salt to taste
4 tablespoons water or white wine
½ cup chopped fresh coriander

1. Steam the peas for 5 minutes and refresh under cold water.

2. Heat the safflower or peanut oil over medium heat in a large, heavy-bottomed frying pan or wok and sauté the mustard seeds and fenugreek seeds for about 10 seconds. Add the ginger and turmeric and stir-fry about 2 minutes, being careful not to allow the ginger to burn (reduce heat if oil is too hot). Add the remaining spices and the sea salt, stir together, then stir in 4 tablespoons water or white wine and mix together well. Add the peas, toss together for a minute or so, and reduce heat. Cover and simmer 15 minutes, or until the peas are tender, checking the liquid every 5 minutes. Add more if necessary.

3. When the peas are tender, stir in the chopped fresh coriander and serve.

Curried Pumpkin–Sweet Potato Purée

Serves 6 to 8

2 pounds fresh pumpkin or winter squash, peeled, seeded, and diced
½ pound sweet potato, baked in its skin until tender
2 tablespoons lime juice
3 tablespoons plain low-fat yogurt, more if needed
2 tablespoons melted butter
1 teaspoon minced or grated fresh ginger, or ¼ teaspoon ground dried
2 teaspoons curry powder
¼ teaspoon cinnamon
Pinch of nutmeg
Sea salt and freshly ground pepper to taste

1. Steam the pumpkin for 15 minutes, or until thoroughly tender. Drain and let drip for a few minutes in a colander.

2. Remove the skin from the baked sweet potato, and purée with the pumpkin in a food processor or through a food mill. Stir in the yogurt and lime juice, and combine well.

3. Melt the butter in a large, heavy-bottomed frying pan or casserole over low heat and add the ginger and curry powder. Cook gently, stirring, for 1 to 2 minutes. Stir in the pumpkin–sweet potato purée, cinnamon, nutmeg, sea salt, and freshly ground pepper, and heat through, stirring. Transfer to a serving dish and serve, or keep warm in a medium oven.

SPICY SAUTÉED ZUCCHINI AND TOMATOES

Serves 4 to 6

1 tablespoon safflower or vegetable oil
1 small onion, chopped
2 cloves garlic, minced or put through a press
2 serrano or jalapeño peppers, seeded and minced
½ teaspoon ground cumin
¼ teaspoon chili powder
1½ pounds zucchini, diced
1 pound tomatoes, seeded and diced
2 tablespoons lemon juice
Sea salt and freshly ground pepper to taste
2 tablespoons chopped fresh coriander

1. Heat the oil in a large, heavy-bottomed frying pan or casserole and add the onion and garlic. Sauté until the onion begins to soften and add the minced peppers, spices, zucchini, and tomatoes. Sauté, stirring, for a couple of minutes (add more oil if necessary), then cover and cook over medium-low heat for 10 to 15 minutes, stirring occasionally.

2. Season to taste with lemon juice, sea salt, and freshly ground pepper. Stir in the coriander and serve.

Louisiana-Style Summer Squash

This spicy, fried dish is a toned-down version of Chef Paul Prudhomme's, from his Louisiana Kitchen *(William Morrow & Co., New York, 1984).*

½ teaspoon sea salt
¾ teaspoon sweet paprika
½ teaspoon ground white pepper
¼ to ½ teaspoon cayenne pepper, to taste
½ teaspoon ground black pepper
¼ teaspoon dried thyme leaves
1½ pounds zucchini or summer squash, cut in rounds
½ cup whole wheat pastry flour
½ cup cornmeal
½ cup milk
1 egg
Safflower or peanut oil for deep-frying

1. Combine the sea salt, spices, and thyme in a small bowl. Sprinkle the diced squash with a teaspoon of the mix.

2. Divide the remaining spice mix in half and stir one half into the flour and the other half into the cornmeal.

3. Beat together the egg and milk.

4. Heat 1 inch of safflower or peanut oil in a deep saucepan or frying pan to 350°F.

5. Using your hands, quickly toss the squash in the flour and shake off any excess flour. Toss in the milk and egg, then dip in the cornmeal to coat. Shake off any excess cornmeal and deep-fry for about 2 minutes. Drain on paper towels and serve at once.

Spicy Okra and Tomato Sauté

Serves 4 to 6

1 tablespoon safflower or vegetable oil
1 large onion, chopped
2 cloves garlic, minced or put through a press
2 teaspoons sweet paprika
1 hot green chili pepper, chopped
1 pound okra, trimmed just below the stem (before the seeds begin) and sliced ¼ to ½ inch thick
1 tablespoon wine vinegar
3 tablespoons white wine
1 pound tomatoes, fresh or canned, sliced
1 tablespoon chopped fresh basil or coriander
Sea salt and freshly ground pepper to taste

1. Heat the oil in a large, heavy-bottomed frying pan or casserole and add the onion and one clove of the garlic. Sauté over medium heat until the onion begins to soften. Add the paprika and chili pepper and continue to sauté another few minutes, stirring.

2. Add the okra and vinegar and sauté until the okra turns bright green, about 5 minutes. Add the wine, tomatoes, and remaining garlic, and cook, stirring from time to time, for 10 to 15 minutes, or until the okra is tender and the mixture aromatic. Add the basil or coriander and season to taste with sea salt and freshly ground pepper. Serve with hot, cooked grains.

Gingered Mushrooms

Serves 4 to 6

1 tablespoon safflower or vegetable oil
1½ pounds mushrooms, cleaned, stems trimmed, cut in halves or quarters if very large
2 shallots, finely chopped
2 cloves garlic, minced or put through a press
2 teaspoons minced or grated fresh ginger
Pinch of cayenne
1 tablespoon soy sauce
2 tablespoons dry white wine
¼ teaspoon thyme
Freshly ground pepper to taste

1. Heat the oil in a large, heavy-bottomed frying pan and add the mushrooms. Sauté for a few minutes, stirring, and add the shallots, garlic, and ginger. Continue to sauté over medium-high heat, stirring, for about 3 minutes.

2. Add the remaining ingredients and continue to cook for another 5 minutes, or until the mushrooms are tender and aromatic. Adjust sea-sonings and serve.

Cucumbers Simmered in White Wine

Serves 4 to 6

1 tablespoon olive or safflower oil
1 onion, thinly sliced
1 teaspoon ground cumin
1 teaspoon curry powder
2 large or 4 small cucumbers, peeled and sliced
Pinch of cayenne
Juice of ½ lemon
1 cup dry white wine
Sea salt and freshly ground pepper to taste
2 tablespoons chopped fresh parsley or coriander

1. Heat the oil in a heavy-bottomed, lidded frying pan or casserole over medium heat and sauté the onion until it begins to soften. Add the cumin and curry powder, stir together, and add the cucumbers. Sauté, stirring, for a minute or two, and add the cayenne, lemon juice, and white wine. Bring to a simmer, reduce heat, cover, and simmer 20 minutes.

2. Uncover pan and turn up the heat. Boil off most of the wine, stirring. Add sea salt and freshly ground pepper to taste, toss with the parsley or fresh coriander, and serve, or chill and serve cold.

Sweet and Sour Red Cabbage with Apples

Serves 4

1 to 2 tablespoons safflower or vegetable oil
1 onion, sliced
1 pound red cabbage, cored and shredded
2 tart apples, peeled, cored and sliced
3 tablespoons apple cider or red wine vinegar
2 tablespoons raisins
½ teaspoon ground cloves
½ teaspoon ground allspice
1 teaspoon ground cinnamon
¼ cup beer or apple juice
2 tablespoons mild-flavored honey
Sea salt to taste
1 cup plain low-fat yogurt

1. Heat 1 tablespoon of the oil in a large, heavy-bottomed frying pan and add the onion. Sauté, stirring, over medium heat until the onion begins to brown, and add the cabbage.

2. Sauté a few minutes (add more oil if necessary) and add the apples, vinegar, raisins, and spices, and stir together well. Add the beer or apple juice and honey, and continue to cook, stirring occasionally, for 10 to 15 minutes.

3. Season to taste with sea salt and freshly ground pepper and remove from the heat. Let cool a moment and stir in the yogurt. Serve at once over hot cooked grains such as bulgur or kasha.

VEGETABLES EN PAPILLOTE WITH GARAM MASALA

Serves 4 to 6

1 pound new potatoes, cut in half or quarters
1 bulb fennel, sliced
1 head garlic, broken into cloves, peeled
8 whole shallots, peeled
1½ tablespoons vegetable oil
Sea salt and freshly ground pepper to taste
1½ teaspoons garam masala (page 27)

1. Prepare a grill or preheat the oven to 375°F.

2. Cut four to six double-thickness squares of aluminum foil, about 12 inches square, and brush with vegetable oil.

3. Toss together the prepared vegetables with the remaining oil, sea salt, freshly ground pepper, and the garam masala. Distribute evenly among the squares of foil.

4. Bring the edges of the foil up around the vegetables and crimp together tightly. Place directly on the coals of the grill or in the preheated oven and bake 45 minutes. Serve directly from the foil.

GINGERED CARROTS

Serves 4 to 6

1½ pounds carrots, peeled and thinly sliced
1 tablespoon butter
⅓ cup fresh orange juice
2 tablespoons mild-flavored honey
1 tablespoons grated orange rind
1 teaspoon grated or minced fresh ginger
¼ teaspoon ground cloves
3 tablespoons red wine

1. Heat the butter in a heavy-bottomed saucepan or casserole. Add the carrots and ginger and sauté for 2 minutes over medium heat.

2. Add the remaining ingredients and bring to a simmer. Cover and simmer 10 minutes.

3. Remove the lid and turn up the heat. Reduce the liquid until it glazes the carrots. Correct seasonings and serve.

Spicy Green Beans

Serves 4 to 6

1½ pounds green beans, ends trimmed
3 tablespoons plain low-fat yogurt
1 teaspoon mild-flavored honey
½ hot, fresh, green chili, thinly sliced
1 teaspoon cornstarch
Sea salt to taste
¾ teaspoon dry English mustard
¾ teaspoon ground cumin
1 tablespoon lemon juice
3 tablespoons safflower or peanut oil
5 whole fenugreek seeds
¼ teaspoon whole cumin
¼ teaspoon garam masala (see page 27)
3 tablespoons chopped fresh coriander

1. Steam the beans for 10 minutes. Drain, refresh under cold water, and slice into thin rounds about ¼ inch thick. Set aside.

2. In a small bowl combine the yogurt, green chili, sea salt, honey, dry mustard, cornstarch, ground cumin, and lemon juice. Add 3 tablespoons water and mix well.

3. Heat the oil in a wide, heavy-bottomed frying pan or wok over medium-high heat. Add the fenugreek, cumin seeds, and garam masala, stir-fry 20 seconds, and add the beans. Cook, tossing, for a minute, then reduce heat to low. Add the yogurt mixture, stir everything together well, cover, and simmer 15 minutes over low heat, stirring from time to time. Stir in the chopped fresh coriander, correct seasonings, and serve with hot, cooked grains.

4
TOFU, GRAINS, LEGUMES, AND PASTAS

DRY COOKED, SPICY TOFU

Use this as a stuffing for vegetables, as a side dish with grains and vegetables, or even as a sandwich filling. It's supposed to have the dry texture and is based on an Indian dish traditionally made with meat.

Serves 4

2 tablespoons safflower or light vegetable oil
1 onion, finely chopped
2 to 3 cloves garlic, to taste, minced or put through a press
1½ tablespoons minced fresh ginger
1 small green chili, seeded and minced
1 pound tofu, diced
2 tablespoons soy sauce
¼ teaspoon turmeric
2 teaspoons garam masala (see page 27)
1 tablespoon lemon juice
2 tablespoons chopped fresh coriander

1. Heat the oil in a wide, heavy-bottomed frying pan and add the onions. Fry over medium heat until beginning to brown, about 5 minutes, stirring constantly.

2. Add the garlic, ginger, and chili, and cook an additional 2 minutes. Add the tofu and mash with the back of your spoon. Add the soy sauce and cook, stirring, until the tofu begins to brown and is quite dry. Add the turmeric, stir for a moment, and stir in the garam masala and lemon juice. The pan will be quite dry, but if you stir quickly the ingredients won't burn. Remove from the heat at once and stir in the coriander. Serve at once or use as a stuffing for vegetables.

Note: This will keep for 2 days in the refrigerator. It does not freeze, however.

Tofu Quiche

Serves 6 to 8

For the Mixed Grains Pie Crust:

½ cup millet meal, made by blending millet in a blender at high speed
¼ cup cornmeal
¾ cup whole wheat pastry flour
¼ teaspoon salt
¼ cup safflower oil
2 to 3 tablespoons cold water
More oil or water if necessary

1. Oil a 9- or 10-inch pie pan or quiche pan. Preheat the oven to 350°F.

2. Mix together the millet meal and cornmeal, and toast it in a dry skillet over medium heat until just beginning to smell toasty. Immediately remove from the heat and place in a mixing bowl. Add the pastry flour and salt, and cut in the oil with a fork or pastry cutter. Add the water and mix thoroughly.

3. This crust won't gather neatly into a ball the way other crusts do, and must be pressed into the pie pan or quiche pan. Pick it up in little pieces and press them piece by piece into the pan, or gather up the mass and press, pressing from the ball of your palm out to your finger-tips. When the pastry bakes, it firms up, so don't worry about the crumbly quality.

4. Prebake the pastry 5 minutes in the oven.

For the Quiche:

1 tablespoon safflower or vegetable oil
1 medium-sized onion, finely chopped
1 to 2 cloves garlic, minced or put through a press
1 teaspoon minced fresh ginger
1½ teaspoons curry powder
1½ pounds tofu

1. Preheat the oven to 350°F.

2. Heat the first tablespoon of oil in a heavy-bottomed frying pan and sauté the onion over medium-low heat with the garlic, minced ginger, and 1 teaspoon of the curry powder until the onion is tender and translucent. Set aside (if using mushrooms, sauté with the onion until tender).

3. Blend all the remaining ingredients (except the optional spinach or broccoli) together in a blender or food processor until completely smooth. Sir in the onion mixture and the optionals. Adjust seasonings, adding more soy sauce, pepper, or curry powder if you wish.

4. Pour the tofu mixture into the prebaked pie crust. Bake at 350°F. for 30 minutes, or until the top begins to brown. Let sit about 10 minutes before serving.

Note: you can also make this quiche without the pastry or bake it in an oiled paté tureen or bread pan and use as a spread.

Optional:
10 ounces spinach, washed, stemmed, blanched, squeezed dry, and chopped OR 2 cups broccoli florets, steamed 5 minutes and coarsely chopped OR 2 cups mushrooms, sliced and sautéed until tender in 1 tablespoon safflower or vegetable oil

2 eggs
½ cup plain low-fat yogurt
⅛ teaspoon cayenne
1 additional tablespoon safflower or sesame oil
⅛ teaspoon freshly ground nutmeg
2 to 3 tablespoons tamari soy sauce, to taste
1 teaspoon lemon juice
2 tablespoons sesame tahini
1 to 2 tablespoons dry sherry, to taste
Freshly ground pepper, to taste

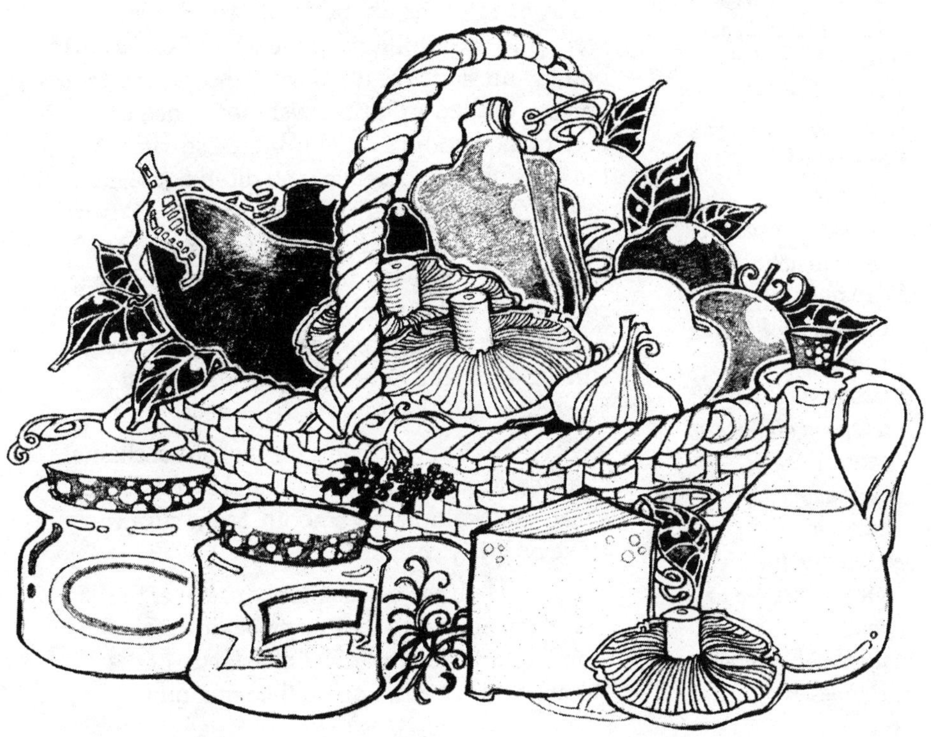

Eggplant Moussaka with Tofu Bechamel

Serves 8 to 10

For the Moussaka:
3 large eggplants
1 tablespoon olive oil
2 additional tablespoons olive oil, safflower oil, or butter
1 large onion, chopped
3 cloves garlic, minced or put through a press
1 cup sliced fresh mushrooms
1 bell pepper, cored, seeded, and diced
3 tomatoes, peeled, seeded, and chopped
½ cup dry white wine
½ to 1 teaspoon thyme, to taste
1 teaspoon oregano, or more to taste
½ cup raw soy grits, cooked, or bulgur, cooked***
½ teaspoon cinnamon
½ teaspoon allspice, or more, to taste
½ cup chopped, fresh parsley
Sea salt and freshly ground pepper to taste
1 cup freshly grated Parmesan

1. Preheat the oven to 450°F. Oil a large baking sheet with olive oil.

2. Slice the eggplants in half lengthwise and score with a sharp knife, being careful not to cut through the skin. Place cut side down on the baking sheet and bake 15 to 20 minutes in the preheated oven, or until the skins begin to shrivel. Meanwhile, prepare the remaining ingredients. Remove the eggplants from the oven, and when cool enough to handle, scoop out the pulp and dice. Reduce the oven heat to 350°F.

3. Heat a large, heavy-bottomed frying pan or wok. Add the additional olive oil, safflower oil, or butter, and sauté the onion with the garlic until the onion is tender. Add the mushrooms, bell pepper, and tomatoes, and sauté 3 minutes, stirring. Add the wine, thyme, oregano, and diced eggplant, and toss together (eggplant will be very soft). Cover and simmer over medium heat for 15 minutes, stirring from time to time. Uncover and stir in the cooked soy grits or bulgur, cinnamon, allspice, parsley, sea salt, and pepper to taste, and cook, stirring another 2 minutes. Taste and adjust seasonings, and remove from the heat.

4. Place all the ingredients for the tofu bechamel in a blender or food processor and blend at high speed until completely smooth. Make sure you leave no gritty chunks.

5. Spread half the eggplant mixture over the bottom of an oiled 11 x 16 inch baking dish or a 4- to 5-quart) casserole. Sprinkle ⅓ cup of the Parmesan over this. Spread the remaining

eggplant mixture over this and sprinkle on another ⅓ cup of the Parmesan. Mix the remaining Parmesan into the tofu bechamel and spread the sauce in a thick layer over the top of the casserole.

6. Bake in the preheated oven for 25 to 30 minutes, or until the top browns.

For the Tofu Bechamel:

1 pound tofu
1 tablespoon dark soy sauce such as tamari or Kikkoman
1½ tablespoons miso paste (a fermented soy paste available in Japanese and natural food stores), or one additional tablespoon soy sauce
½ cup plain low-fat yogurt
¼ cup water
1 teaspoon minced fresh ginger
3 tablespoons sesame tahini
3 tablespoons dry sherry
1 tablespoon lemon juice
Pinch of freshly grated nutmeg
Small pinch of cayenne

**To cook the soy grits, combine with 2 cups water in a heavy saucepan and bring to a boil. Reduce the heat and simmer, covered, for 50 minutes. Add sea salt to taste and drain off excess water.*

***To cook the bulgur, place in a bowl and pour on 1 cup of boiling water. Let sit 20 to 30 minutes, until fluffy. Drain off excess water. Add sea salt to taste.*

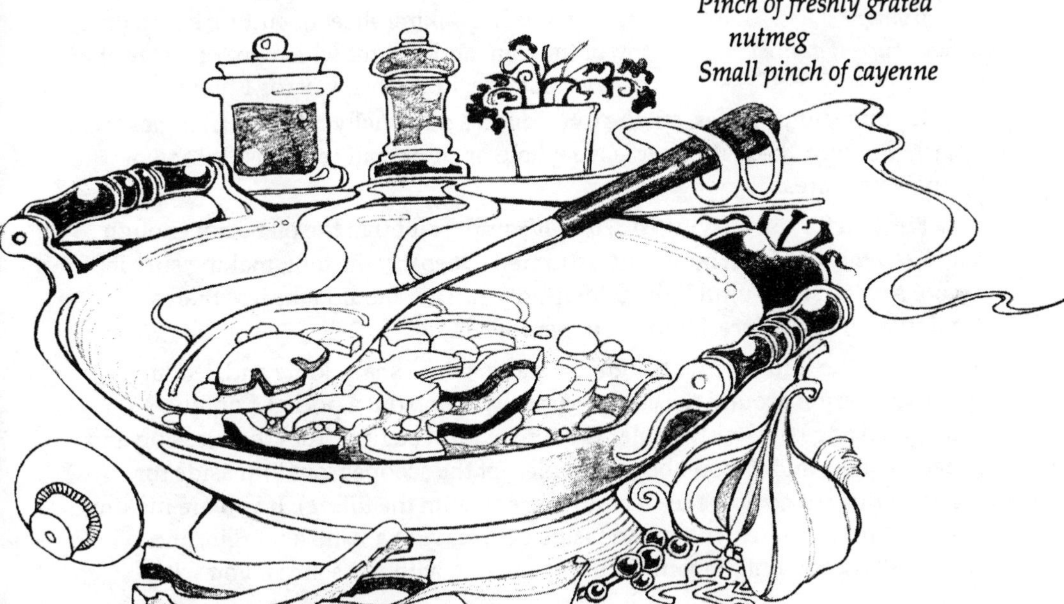

Stuffed Tofu Pockets, Squares, or Triangles

This is one of the most convenient and intriguing ways to serve bean curd. You press 12-ounce squares, cut them into two large triangles or squares, and deep-fry the pressed tofu. This gives it a tough outer skin and renders it almost like chicken. Then you scoop out the insides and stuff the hollowed-out shell as if it were pita bread. Or you can leave the tofu in the shape of a square and scoop out the middle so that it's like a box. A number of fillings will work. In addition to the delicious suggestions below, the pressed, deep-fried tofu makes a great container for leftovers.

Serving tofu this way increases the protein content of your meal tremendously. A pressed 12-ounce square is not much more filling than a 4-ounce piece, the usual serving, but it has three times as much protein.

One thing that's great about these is that they keep for a longer time than fresh, unpressed tofu. Once pressed and deep-fried, they needn't be covered with water; just keep them in the refrigerator in a covered container. They will hold for up to three days this way; and if you have them on hand, you can have marvelous stuffed tofu dinners in minutes.

Serves 4

4 12-ounce squares tofu
1 quart safflower or vegetable oil, for deep-frying
Soy sauce, if desired

1. Trim the tofu into neat 12-ounce squares and wrap in a dish towel. Cover a baking sheet with two layers of paper towels and place the tofu on top. Set another baking sheet or cutting board on top of the tofu, and weight with a pot of water or a heavy casserole. Press this way for 1 hour.

2. If you want triangles, cut the tofu squares diagonally into two triangles each. For tofu "boxes" either leave whole or cut in half crosswise into two smaller squares.

3. Heat oil for deep-frying to 370°F. It's important that the oil be hot enough to keep the tofu from becoming saturated. Deep-fry the tofu, making sure it cooks on all sides, until light golden-brown. This should take less than a minute for each piece. Drain on paper towels.

4. When the tofu is cool enough to handle, take a sharp knife and, leaving a ¼-inch margin around the edges, carefully scoop out a pocket from the diagonal edge of your triangle. The tofu should be firm from the pressing and deep-frying, and it won't be too fragile. Set the scooped-out tofu aside for another use (it could be used as an ingredient in the filling). If you are making stuffed tofu squares, cut out an inside box, leaving a ¼-inch margin, and carefully scoop out the tofu. Douse the inside with soy sauce if you wish.

5. You should be able to get about ¼ cup of filling into the triangles and more into the squares. Hold the deep-fried tofu in the refrig-erator until ready to fill, or hold the filled triangles or squares in the refrigerator until ready to serve. These can be served cold, at room temperature, or hot. To serve hot, heat through in a 325°F. oven for 20 minutes.

Variation I

Heat the oil in a wok or heavy-bottomed frying pan and sauté the onion until just about tender. Add the carrots, cashews, tofu, and ginger, and sauté about 3 minutes. Add the soy sauce, chili pepper, and cucumber, and sauté about 2 minutes. Add the Pernod and coriander, sauté another 1 or 2 minutes, and remove from the heat. Hold until ready to fill the tofu pockets.

Variation II

1. Toss together the beansprouts, radishes, cucumber, walnuts, and coriander leaves.

2. Place the remaining ingredients in a blender and blend together at high speed until smooth. Toss with the vegetables. Hold until ready to fill the tofu. This will keep for a day or two in the refrigerator.

Notes: Both filling recipes yield enough for 8 stuffed pockets. You could also serve these fillings as salads.

Variation II Hot-and-Sour Beansprouts Filling:

2 cups mung beansprouts, coarsely chopped
3 radishes, sliced
½ cucumber, peeled and shredded
¼ cup chopped walnuts
2 tablespoons chopped fresh coriander
2 tablespoons crunchy peanut butter
1 tablespoon dark soy sauce such as tamari or Kikkoman
2 tablespoons cider or white wine vinegar
½ teaspoon hot red pepper powder or hot pepper oil
1½ teaspoons sesame oil
1 tablespoon safflower oil
2 teaspoons freshly grated or minced ginger
1 clove garlic, peeled
½ cup vegetable stock (page 54) or bouillon

Variation I
Cashew Carrot Filling:

1 tablespoon sesame or safflower oil
1 small onion, minced
1½ cups julienned carrots
¾ cup cashews
¾ cup scooped-out tofu from the squares
1 teaspoon finely minced or grated fresh ginger (more to taste)
1 tablespoon dark soy sauce, such as tamari or Kikkoman
1 small, hot, dried red chilli pepper, minced, or ½ teaspoon hot pepper oil, available in Oriental markets
½ cup shredded cucumber
1 tablespoon Pernod or anise-flavored liqueur
3 tablespoons chopped fresh coriander

CURRIED TOFU AND VEGETABLES

Serves 6 to 8

2 tablespoons butter
1 tablespoon peanut or safflower oil
1 teaspoon mustard seeds
1 teaspoon cumin seeds, crushed
½ teaspoon turmeric
½ teaspoon chili powder
2 to 3 teaspoons curry powder, to taste
1 medium onion, sliced
1 clove garlic, minced or put through a press
1 teaspoon minced fresh ginger
½ pound tofu, pressed if desired (see page 109) and diced
½ pound zucchini, sliced
1 pound cauliflower, broken into florets and sliced
½ pound yellow squash, sliced
¼ cup raw peanuts, almonds, or sunflower seeds
½ cup raisins
¼ cup water or vegetable stock
Sea salt and freshly ground pepper to taste
1 tablespoon cornstarch or arrowroot dissolved in 1½ tablespoons water
1 cup plain low-fat yogurt
2 tablespoons chopped fresh coriander

1. Heat the butter and oil together in a large, heavy-bottomed frying pan, casserole, or wok, and add the spices, onion, garlic, and ginger. Sauté until the onion is tender, and add the tofu. Sauté gently over a medium-low flame for 5 minutes, and add the zucchini, cauliflower, and squash. Cook, stirring, for 5 minutes. Add the raisins, nuts, and water or stock, cover, and simmer 5 to 10 minutes. Add sea salt and freshly ground pepper to taste, adjust seasonings, and stir in the dissolved cornstarch or arrowroot. Cook, stirring, until the vegetables are glazed, and remove from the heat.

2. Transfer to a serving dish and stir in the yogurt. Serve at once over hot, cooked grains, or with one of the pilafs on pages 110, 111, 112, 113.

Tempura'd Tofu

Serves 4 to 6

For the Tofu:

*1½ pounds pressed tofu**
½ cup dark soy sauce such as tamari or Kikkoman
¼ cup water
1 clove garlic, crushed
1 teaspoon minced fresh ginger
½ teaspoon cinnamon
¼ teaspoon ground allspice
¼ teaspoon crushed anise or fennel seeds
⅛ teaspoon ground cloves
¼ to ½ cup whole wheat pastry flour, as needed
1 quart safflower or vegetable oil, for deep-frying

For the Batter:

½ teaspoon sea salt
1 cup sifted whole wheat pastry flour, or a combination of whole wheat pastry and unbleached white flour
2 tablespoons safflower, sesame or vegetable oil
2 eggs, separated
1 cup water

1. Make the batter. Combine the flour, salt, oil, egg yolks, and water. Stir together but don't beat. Let stand for 20 minutes while you simmer the tofu (see Step 2). Then whip the egg whites until fluffy but not stiff, and fold them into the batter.

2. While the batter is resting, combine the soy sauce, water, garlic, ginger, and spices in a saucepan and bring to a simmer. Cut the pressed tofu into slivers ¼ to ½ inch wide and simmer in the soy sauce mixture for 15 minutes. Remove with a slotted spoon and drain. Retain the soy sauce for dipping.

3. Slowly heat the oil in a saucepan, wok, or deep-fryer to 370°F. It is important to get the oil to this temperature before attempting to deep-fry and to maintain the temperature throughout.

4. Carefully dredge the tofu in the flour, then dip into the batter. Deep-fry until golden brown and drain on paper towels. Arrange on a platter with other vegetables, garnish with parsley or fresh coriander, and serve with the simmering liquid.

**To press tofu for tempuras and stir-fries: Cut tofu into 4-ounce squares and wrap in a dish cloth. Place two layers of paper towel on a baking sheet and set the tofu on top. Set a cutting board or another baking sheet on top of the tofu, and weight that with a 3- to 4-quart saucepan filled with water, or a heavy casserole. Press for an hour. Refrigerate wrapped in a wet towel, if not using right away. Pressed tofu stays together better than unpressed tofu when you cook it and has an almost chicken-like texture.*

NORTH INDIAN PILAF

This recipe is adapted from Julie Sahni's "Patiala Pilaf."

Serves 6 to 8

2 cups basmati rice
4 cups cold water
2 tablespoons vegetable oil
1 onion, chopped
2 cloves garlic, minced or put through a press
6 green cardamom pods
1 cinnamon stick, 3 inches long
8 whole cloves
½ teaspoon powdered ginger
2 bay leaves
1 teaspoon sea salt

1. Wash the rice thoroughly in several rinses of cold water. Soak in the cold water for 30 minutes. Drain and retain the soaking liquid.

2. Heat the oil in a large, lidded frying pan or wok and sauté the onion until tender. Add the garlic and sauté 1 minute, then add the spices and sauté another 30 seconds, stirring.

3. Add the rice and more oil if necessary, and sauté, stirring, over moderate heat, until translucent and beginning to brown. Add the soaking liquid, sea salt, and bay leaves. Bring to a boil, stirring, then reduce heat and partially cover. Simmer 10 to 12 minutes, or until most of the water has evaporated and there are small steam holes covering the surface of the rice.

4. Now cover the rice tightly and place the pan or wok on a wok ring, a flame-tamer, or a heat-resistant pad. Turn heat very low and continue to cook for 10 minutes, undisturbed. Turn off heat and allow rice to sit, undisturbed, another 5 minutes. Turn out onto a warm platter, surround with one of the vegetable dishes in Chapter 3, and serve.

Note: The whole spices are not meant to be eaten but will do no harm if they are.

Sweet Saffron Pilaf with Fruit

Serves 6 to 8

2 cups basmati rice
4 cups water
1 teaspoon saffron threads
2 tablespoons safflower or vegetable oil
10 whole cloves
8 green cardamom pods
1 3-inch stick cinnamon
½ cup dark or golden raisins
½ cup chopped dried apricots
2 tablespoons honey
1 teaspoon sea salt
4 tablespoons slivered blanched almonds
4 ripe peaches, blanched, peeled, and sliced

1. Wash the basmati rice thoroughly in several rinses of cold water. Place in a bowl and soak in the water for 30 minutes. Drain and retain the soaking water.

2. Meanwhile crumble the saffron threads by mashing between your fingers or with the back of a spoon. Add two tablespoons warm water and continue to mash until the threads are dissolved.

3. Heat the safflower oil in a large, lidded frying pan or wok and sauté the spices over medium heat for about 30 seconds. Add the drained rice and sauté, stirring, until the rice is translucent and beginning to toast. Add the liquid which you set aside, the saffron, raisins, dried apricots, honey, and sea salt. Bring to a boil, stirring, then reduce heat, cover partially, and simmer 10 to 12 minutes, or until most of the water is absorbed and there are little steam holes in the surface of the rice.

4. Meanwhile brown the almonds in a little butter or in no butter, either in a dry frying pan or in a moderate oven. Set aside with the sliced peaches.

5. Now cover tightly and place your pan or wok either on a wok ring or on a flame-tamer or heat-resistant pad and turn the heat very low. Steam the pilaf, undisturbed, for 10 minutes. Turn off the heat and let sit without disturbing for another 5 minutes.

6. Transfer the pilaf to a warm platter, sprinkle the top with almonds, and sliced peaches, and serve.

Note: The whole spices aren't meant to be eaten but won't harm you if they are.

Wheat Berry and Soy Pilaf

Serves 4 to 6

3 cups vegetable stock (page 54) or bouillon
2 tablespoons safflower or vegetable oil
1 clove garlic, minced or put through a press
½ medium-sized onion, minced
2 teaspoons grated or minced fresh ginger
½ pound mushrooms, cleaned, trimmed, and sliced
1 teaspoon cumin seeds
1 cup whole wheat berries
½ cup soy flakes
½ cup dry white wine or beer
Sea salt and freshly ground pepper to taste
½ pound broccoli florets or zucchini, sliced
2 tablespoons chopped fresh parsley

1. Have the stock simmering in a saucepan.

2. In a large, heavy-bottomed, lidded casserole heat 1 tablespoon of the oil and sauté the garlic and onion until the onion begins to soften. Add the ginger, mushrooms, and cumin seeds, and continue to sauté another 3 minutes.

3. Add a little more oil and the wheat berries and soy flakes. Sauté, stirring, until the grains separate and begin to smell toasty, about 2 minutes. Add the wine or beer and cook, stirring, over medium heat until the liquid has just about been absorbed.

4. Add the stock or bouillon, stirring, and bring to a boil. Cover, reduce heat, and simmer 45 minutes, checking after 30 minutes to make sure there is still enough liquid. Add more if the mixture seems dry or near-dry.

5. Add the broccoli or zucchini, salt and freshly ground pepper to taste, and cover. Steam the vegetables with the grains for 5 to 10 minutes, to taste.

6. When the grains and vegetables are tender, pour off any excess cooking liquid, toss with the parsley, and serve.

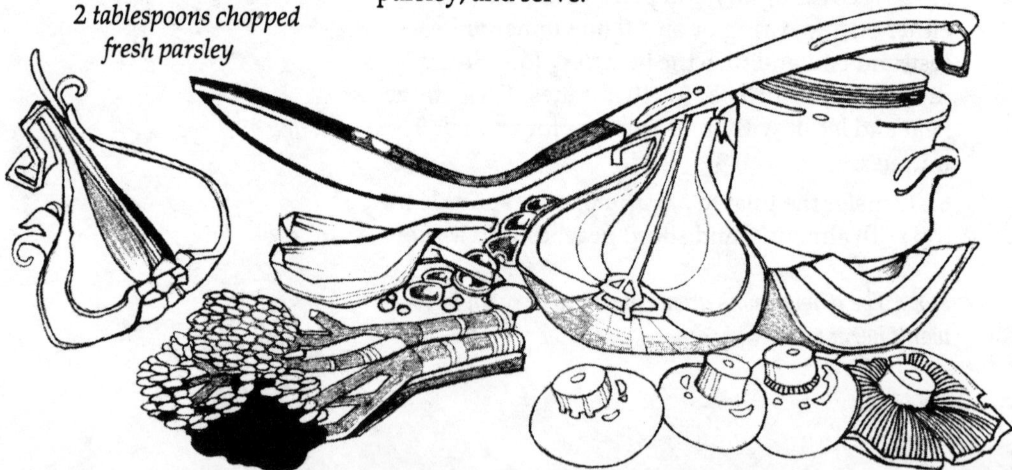

BROCCOLI AND CASHEW PILAF

Serves 6 to 8

1 cup raw cashews
2 tablespoons safflower or vegetable oil
2 teaspoons cumin seeds
1 small onion, minced
2 cloves garlic, minced or put through a press
2 teaspoons minced or grated fresh ginger
1 bunch broccoli, separated into florets, stems peeled and sliced 1/4 inch thick
2 1/2 cups cooked brown rice or basmati rice
1 teaspoon Mughal garam masala (page 26)
Sea salt to taste
2 oranges, peeled, white pith removed, and cut in rounds

1. Roast the cashews in a dry frying pan or a moderate oven until light brown. Set aside.

2. Heat the oil in a large, lidded frying pan or wok and add the cumin. Sauté over medium heat for about 20 seconds, stirring, then add the onion, garlic, and ginger. Sauté, stirring, until the onion is tender, and add the broccoli. Sauté, stirring, for about 2 minutes, and add 1/3 cup of water. Bring to a simmer, cover, and simmer 8 to 10 minutes over medium-low heat, or until the broccoli is just tender.

3. Stir in the rice, cashews, and Mughal garam masala and add sea salt to taste. Heat through, stirring, for about 5 minutes. Transfer to a warm platter, garnish with the oranges, and serve.

"Dirty" Rice

Serves 4 to 6

For the Beans:

1 cup red beans, washed, picked over, and soaked
1 onion, chopped
3 cloves garlic, minced or put through a press
3 cups water
1 teaspoon sea salt
1 bay leaf

For the Rice:

¾ teaspoon cayenne pepper
½ teaspoon sea salt (more or less to taste)
1 teaspoon ground black pepper
1¼ teaspoons sweet paprika
1 teaspoon dry mustard
1 teaspoon ground cumin
½ teaspoon dried thyme
½ teaspoon oregano
2 tablespoons safflower oil
1 additional onion, chopped
3 large cloves garlic, minced or put through a press
1 stalk celery, chopped
1 green pepper, chopped
1 cup brown rice
2 cups cooking liquid from the beans
1 cup water

1. First cook the beans. Combine all the ingredients for the beans except the sea salt in a large soup pot or casserole and bring to a boil. Reduce heat, cover, and simmer 2 hours, or until the beans are tender, adding the salt halfway through. Drain, remove the bay leaf and set aside ¾ pint (2 cups) of the cooking liquid (add water to make up the amount if there isn't that much).

2. Combine all the spices and herbs for the dirty rice in a small bowl.

3. Heat the safflower oil over medium-low heat in a large, heavy-bottomed casserole and add the onion and garlic. Sauté until the onion begins to soften and add the celery and green pepper. Continue to sauté, stirring, another minute or two and add the spice mixture. Sauté, stirring constantly, over medium-low heat for about 30 seconds, then add the rice, the beans, and bean liquid you set aside, and the water. Bring to a boil, reduce heat, cover, and simmer 30 to 45 minutes, or until the rice is cooked al dente and most of the liquid absorbed (it can be a little soupy). Serve in bowls.

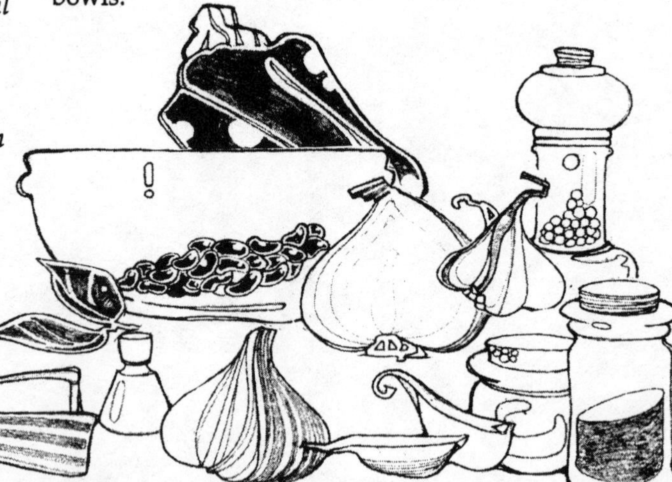

Indian Fried Rice

Serves 6 to 8

2 tablespoons safflower or vegetable oil
1 onion, chopped
2 cloves garlic, minced or put through a press
1 teaspoon minced fresh ginger
1 small head cauliflower or broccoli, broken into florets, stems peeled and sliced ¼ inch thick
2 carrots, peeled and sliced thin
2½ cups cooked brown rice or basmati rice
2 teaspoons ground roasted cumin seeds
1 teaspoon ground roasted coriander
1 teaspoon Mughal garam masala (page 26)
Sea salt to taste
3 tablespoons chopped fresh coriander

1. Heat the oil over medium heat in a large, heavy-bottomed, lidded frying pan or wok and stir-fry the onion, garlic, and ginger until the onion is tender. Add the remaining vegetables and stir-fry about 3 minutes, or until lightly browned. Add 6 tablespoons of cold water, cover, and simmer for 5 minutes over medium-low heat, or until the vegetables are cooked through but still somewhat crunchy.

2. Add the rice, sea salt to taste, and spices. Mix together well, and cover and cook over low heat for 5 minutes. Stir from time to time. (A thin layer of rice will probably stick to the bottom; it will detach easily with soaking.) Correct seasonings, stir in the fresh coriander, and serve.

Spanish Rice

Serves 6

1 quart simmering vegetable stock (page 54)
1 tablespoon butter or safflower oil
½ onion, minced
2 large cloves garlic, minced or put through a press
1 teaspoon sweet paprika
1½ cups brown rice
1 green bell pepper, cut in thin strips
3 tomatoes, seeded and chopped
¼ cup dry white wine
½ teaspoon saffron
1 cup fresh peas
Sea salt and freshly ground pepper to taste

1. Have the stock simmering in a saucepan.

2. Heat the butter or oil in a large, heavy-bottomed, lidded frying pan or casserole and add the onion and garlic. Cook, stirring, until the onion is tender. Add the paprika and the rice and cook, stirring, for 1 minute. Add the pepper and tomatoes and stir together for a couple of minutes.

3. Add the wine and continue to stir until the liquid is absorbed. Add the simmering stock and the saffron, bring to a second boil, cover, and reduce heat. Simmer for 30 minutes. Add the peas and continue to cook until all the liquid is absorbed or until the rice is cooked al dente and the peas cooked through, about 10 more minutes. Pour off any stock that remains, correct seasonings, and serve.

Sweet Couscous

Serves 8 generously

2 cups couscous
3 cups water
1¼ cups raisins
Boiling water to cover
2 tablespoons butter
1 onion, chopped
4 tablespoons slivered blanched almonds
½ cup chopped dried apricots
2 tablespoons cinnamon
½ teaspoon turmeric
1 teaspoon ground ginger
Sea salt to taste
3 tablespoons honey
2 oranges, peeled, white membranes removed, chopped

1. Place the couscous in a bowl and pour on the water. Let sit while you prepare the remaining ingredients.

2. Place the raisins in a bowl and pour on boiling water to cover. Let sit 15 minutes, then drain and retain the soaking water. Add water to measure 2 cups.

3. Heat the butter in a heavy-bottomed, lidded saucepan, or in the bottom of a couscoussière. Sauté the onion over medium-low heat until it begins to turn golden. Add the raisins, almonds, dried apricots, spices, honey, and soaking liquid from the raisins. Cover and simmer 25 to 30 minutes.

4. Meanwhile rub the couscous between the palms of your hands, then place in the top part of the couscoussière or in a steamer above the simmering sauce and steam 25 to 30 minutes. Transfer to a platter and toss with the sweet, spicy sauce and the oranges. Serve at once.

FALAFEL

Serves 6 to 8

For the Croquettes:

1 cup garbanzos, washed, picked over, and soaked
Sea salt to taste
¼ cup lemon juice
¼ cup plain low-fat yogurt
2 large cloves garlic
6 heaping tablespoons sesame tahini
½ teaspoon baking soda
1 teaspoon ground cumin
½ teaspoon ground coriander (more to taste)
½ cup whole wheat pastry flour
½ cup sesame seeds
¼ teaspoon sea salt
2 eggs
Safflower or peanut oil for deep-frying

For the Rest of the Falafel:

6 to 8 whole wheat pita breads
3 ripe tomatoes, chopped
1 small onion, chopped
1 small cucumber, chopped
½ cup chopped fresh parsley
1 clove garlic, minced or put through a press
Juice of 1 large lemon
Ground cayenne to taste
¼ teaspoon chili powder
Sea salt and freshly ground pepper to taste

For the Yogurt-Tahini Spread:

½ cup plain low-fat yogurt
3 tablespoons sesame tahini
Juice of ½ lemon
1 clove garlic, minced or put through a press
Sea salt to taste
Pinch of cayenne
Additional hot sauce (optional)

1. Cook the beans in salted water until tender. Drain and purée with sea salt to taste, the lemon juice, yogurt, garlic, baking soda, cumin, and coriander. Let rest for 30 minutes. Meanwhile prepare the other ingredients. Chop the tomatoes, onion, cucumber, and parsley and toss together with the garlic, lemon juice, and spices. Season to taste with sea salt and freshly ground pepper. Set aside.

2. Roll the purée into balls about 2 inches in diameter, and set aside.

3. Start oil heating in a deep pan or wok. Mix together the flour and sesame seeds in a bowl or on a plate. Beat the eggs in another bowl.

4. Dip the garbanzo balls into the egg, then coat lightly with the flour-sesame mixture and deep-fry in the oil until golden brown. Drain on paper towels. Keep warm in a low oven.

5. Mix together the ingredients for the yogurt sauce. Cut the pita breads in half and spoon a little sauce into each half. Place a few balls in each half and top with the vegetable mixture. Serve with additional hot sauce on the side if you wish.

SPICED YELLOW MUNG BEANS

This is adapted from Julie Sahni's recipe.

Serves 4

1 cup yellow mung beans, washed and picked over
1 small onion, chopped
2 cloves garlic, minced or put through a press
1 tablespoon safflower or vegetable oil
¼ teaspoon turmeric
½ teaspoon grated fresh ginger
1 teaspoon sea salt
2 tablespoons additional safflower or vegetable oil
½ teaspoon black mustard seeds
1 green chili, seeded and chopped
1 tablespoon lemon juice
2 tablespoons chopped fresh coriander

1. Heat 1 tablespoon of oil over medium heat in a large, heavy-bottomed casserole and sauté the onion and garlic until the onion is tender. Add the beans, ginger, turmeric, sea salt, and 4 cups water. Bring to a boil, stirring, reduce heat, and simmer 30 minutes, stirring occasionally, or until the beans are tender. Mash the beans to a purée with the back of your spoon or with a wire whisk.

2. Heat the remaining oil in a frying pan over medium heat and add the mustard seeds. Stir a few seconds, or until they turn gray and stop sputtering, and add the chili pepper. Stir for a moment, then stir into the bean purée along with the lemon juice and chopped fresh coriander. Correct seasonings and serve.

Note: This will keep for 2 to 3 days in a refrigerator and freezes well.

Garbanzo Bean Curry

Serves 6

1 to 2 tablespoons safflower or vegetable oil
1 cup thinly sliced onion
1 cup thinly sliced carrot
2 large cloves garlic, minced or put through a press
1½ tablespoons curry powder
1 teaspoon garam masala (see page 27)
2 tomatoes, peeled and chopped
1 pound garbanzos, cooked (save liquid)
Pinch of cayenne
Sea salt and freshly ground pepper to taste
1 to 2 tablespoons fresh lime juice, to taste
1 tablespoon fresh chopped coriander

1. Heat 1 tablespoon safflower oil in a large, heavy-bottomed skillet or wok over low heat and stir in the onion, garlic, ginger, and spices. Cook gently for a few minutes and add the carrot. Continue to cook, stirring, until the onion is tender. Add more oil if necessary. Stir in the tomatoes, garbanzos, enough of the reserved cooking liquid to cover them, cayenne, and salt and freshly ground pepper to taste. Stir well and mash slightly with the back of a spoon.

2. Cook over medium heat for about 10 to 15 minutes, stirring from time to time, or until the beans are quite thick. Remove from the heat, add the lime juice and coriander, and serve.

Sour Lentil Dahl

Serves 6

1½ cups pink or regular lentils, washed, picked over
1 tablespoon chopped fresh ginger
5 cups water
½ teaspoon turmeric
A 1-inch ball of tamarind
1 cup boiling water
1 teaspoon sea salt
2 tablespoons safflower or vegetable oil
1 teaspoon cumin seeds
3 cloves garlic, minced or put through a press
¼ teaspoon cayenne, more to taste

1. Combine the lentils, ginger, turmeric, and 5 cups water in a large saucepan or casserole and bring to a boil. Stir for a minute, reduce heat, cover, and simmer 25 to 30 minutes, or until the lentils are soft.

2. Meanwhile place the tamarind in a small bowl and pour on 1 cup of boiling water. Allow to soak for 15 minutes, then mash with the back of a wooden spoon or your fingers. Strain, pressing all the fibers against the strainer to extract all the juice, and add the liquid to the lentils along with the sea salt.

3. Remove the cooked lentils from the heat and beat to a purée with a whisk or spoon (you can also thicken by puréeing 1 or 2 cups in a blender). Measure out 6 cups, adding water if necessary. Correct salt.

4. Heat the safflower oil in a small frying pan and add the cumin seeds, garlic, and cayenne. Sauté over medium-low heat just until the garlic is tender. Do not brown. Quickly stir into the lentil dahl and mix together well. Heat through, stirring, and serve.

Ginger-Flavored Buckwheat Pasta

Serves 4 to 6

½ cup buckwheat flour
1 cup whole wheat pastry or unbleached white flour
2 teaspoons ground ginger
¼ to ½ teaspoon sea salt, to taste
2 eggs
1 teaspoon sesame oil

1. *Using a food processor:* Place the flours, ginger, and salt in the bowl of your food processor fit-ted with the steel blade and pulse several times to blend together. Add the eggs and sesame oil and process until the mixture is well blended. Take up the dough and press together, then knead for about 10 minutes by squeezing the dough from end to end, passing it from one hand to the other, or by slamming it down on a work surface, squeezing it, taking it up, and slamming it down again. Dough will be soft and you may need to flour your hands a little bit. Wrap the dough in a plastic wrap and let rest for 30 minutes (dough can also be refrigerated at this point for a day or two, tightly wrapped in plastic).

2. *Mixing the dough by hand:* Sift together the flours, salt, and ginger. Place on your work surface in a mound, then make a well in the center. Break the eggs in the well and add the sesame oil. Gently beat the eggs together with a fork. Now begin brushing flour from the edges of the well into the eggs and incorporate in as much as you can with the fork. Use one hand to brush in the flour and to keep building up the edges of the well so that the eggs don't run out while you beat with the other. When most of the flour has been incorporated, gather up the dough and knead together. Brush away all the little balls of flour and egg which remain on the work surface. Knead the dough and proceed as above.

3. Roll out the dough by using a pasta roller or a rolling pin. Cut fettucine or spaghetti noodles, dust lightly with flour, and cook until al dente.

Fresh, they will cook in 30 seconds. These can also be dried or frozen. Dust fairly generously so they don't stick together. They will keep in the refrigerator for several days. If you freeze them, transfer directly from the freezer to boiling water to cook.

Spicy Soba

Serves 4 to 6

Bring a large pot of water to a boil and add the safflower or vegetable oil and the sea salt. Add the noodles and cook until al dente, about 4 to 5 minutes. Drain and toss immediately with the remaining ingredients. Serve hot or cold.

¾ pound buckwheat noodles or ginger-flavored buckwheat pasta (page 122)
1 tablespoon safflower or vegetable oil
2 teaspoons sea salt
3 tablespoons sesame oil
½ to 1 teaspoon hot Chinese red pepper flakes or powder, to taste
1 tablespoon soy sauce

Syrian Lentils with Noodles

Serves 6 to 8

2 tablespoons safflower or vegetable oil
1 onion, chopped
2 to 3 cloves garlic, to taste, minced or put through a press
2 teaspoons ground roasted cumin
1 teaspoon ground roasted coriander
1 to 2 small cayenne peppers, to taste
2 cups lentils, washed and picked over
1 bay leaf
7 cups water
Sea salt and freshly ground pepper to taste
4 ounces broken whole wheat spaghetti noodles, vermicelli, or macaroni

1. Heat the oil in a large, heavy-bottomed casserole and sauté the onion with the garlic until the onion is tender. Add the cumin and coriander and continue to sauté another minute or so over medium heat.

2. Add the cayenne pepper, lentils, bay leaf, and water, and bring to a boil. Add sea salt and pepper to taste, cover, reduce heat, and simmer 45 minutes, or until the lentils are tender. Adjust seasonings.

3. Shortly before serving bring to a simmer and add the noodles. Cook until al dente (4 to 10 minutes depending on the kind of noodle) and serve at once in bowls.

5
DAIRY AND EGGS

BAKED TUNISIAN EGGAH

Serves 4 to 6

3 tablespoons olive oil
4 cloves garlic, thinly sliced
1 onion, thinly sliced
1 sweet green pepper, seeded and thinly sliced
1 sweet red pepper, seeded and thinly sliced
2 zucchini, sliced about ¼ inch thick
1 pound ripe tomatoes, peeled and cut in wedges
¼ to ½ teaspoon cayenne pepper, to taste
¾ teaspoon ground cumin
½ teaspoon ground coriander
½ teaspoon cinnamon
Sea salt and freshly ground pepper to taste
4 tablespoons chopped fresh parsley
6 eggs

1. Heat the olive oil in a large, heavy-bottomed, lidded frying pan or casserole and add the onion and garlic. Sauté gently until the onion begins to soften. Add the green and red peppers and continue to sauté another 5 minutes, stirring. Add the zucchini and continue to sauté another 5 minutes. Stir in the tomatoes, spices, and sea salt and freshly ground pepper to taste. Stir together, cover, and reduce heat. Simmer gently for 30 to 40 minutes, or until the vegetables are cooked through and fragrant. If they begin to stick to the bottom of the pan, add a little water. Correct seasonings and remove from the heat.

2. Meanwhile preheat the oven to 350°F, and oil or butter a baking dish large enough to accommodate the vegetables and eggs.

3. Beat the eggs in a large bowl and add the parsley. Stir in the vegetable mixture, correct seasonings again, and turn into the prepared baking dish. Cover and bake 30 minutes. Remove the cover and bake another 10 minutes, or until the top is nicely browned and the eggs set. Serve at once.

Notes: You could also allow this to cool and serve, cut in squares, as an appetizer.

Scrambled Eggs with Hot Tomato Sauce

Serves 6 to 8

2 tablespoons safflower or vegetable oil
1 onion, finely chopped
3 cloves garlic, minced or put through a press
1 tablespoon finely minced fresh ginger
1 hot green chili, minced, or ¼ teaspoon cayenne
1 3-inch stick cinnamon
8 green or white cardamom pods
2 teaspoons ground coriander
½ teaspoon turmeric
1 pound tomatoes, peeled and finely chopped
1 teaspoon garam masala (see page 27)
¼ teaspoon freshly ground black pepper
Sea salt to taste
8 eggs
3 tablespoons chopped fresh coriander

1. Heat the oil in a large, heavy-bottomed frying pan and add the onion, garlic, and ginger. Sauté over medium heat until the onion is tender. Add the hot chili or cayenne, the cinnamon stick, cardamom, coriander, and turmeric, and stir together. Sauté about a minute and add the tomatoes, garam masala, and pepper. Cook, stirring often, over medium heat for 20 minutes. Add sea salt to taste and correct seasonings. Turn heat very low.

2. Beat the eggs in a bowl and stir in the coriander. Stir into the tomato sauce and cook gently, stirring all the while, until set. Serve at once.

Note: The hot tomato sauce can also be used as an omelet filling, or it can be mixed with the eggs and the whole cooked as an eggah or Spanish omelet.

Curried Walnut and Apple Omelet

Serves 4

1 tart apple, thinly sliced
1 tablespoon butter
1 teaspoon curry powder
½ teaspoon turmeric
¼ teaspoon ground ginger
6 eggs
¾ cup chopped walnuts
Sea salt and freshly ground pepper to taste

1. Heat the butter in a wide omelet pan or frying pan and add the apple, curry powder, turmeric, and ginger. Sauté gently for about 5 minutes.

2. Beat the eggs in a bowl and stir in the walnuts, sea salt, and freshly ground pepper to taste. Add to the pan and tilt the pan so that the egg spreads out in an even layer. Cook over medium-low heat, gently lifting the edges of the omelet and tilting the pan to let the eggs run under-neath until the eggs are just about set, about 5 minutes.

3. Place the omelet under the broiler for a few minutes, or until the top of the omelet puffs and is cooked through. Serve at once, cut in wedges.

Puffed Yogurt Omelet

This simple dish puffs up like a soufflé, and you don't even have to separate the eggs. It is intriguingly simple and has a very delicate flavor and texture.

Serves 3 to 4

6 eggs
1 cup plain low-fat yogurt
½ teaspoon curry powder
1 to 2 small fresh green chilies, seeded and minced (optional)
Sea salt to taste
1 tablespoon butter
½ teaspoon ground roasted cumin (see page 7)
1 tablespoon chopped fresh coriander

1. Beat together the eggs, yogurt, curry powder, optional chilies, and sea salt to taste.

2. Heat the butter over medium-high heat in a 9- or 10-inch, preferably non-stick, frying pan or omelet pan. When the butter stops sizzling, pour in the eggs. Swirl the pan to coat evenly. Keep swirling for about 30 seconds while you gently lift the edges of the omelet, allowing the eggs to run underneath.

3. Now sprinkle the top with the ground roasted cumin and the fresh coriander and turn the heat down to very low. Cover the pan with a lid or another pan turned upside down, and do not disturb for 5 to 7 minutes.

4. Uncover the pan (the omelet should be puffed; cook another few minutes if it is still uncooked on top) and bring to the table at once. Slice in wedges and serve.

Steve's Migas

Serves 6

1. Beat the eggs lightly in a large bowl. Add sea salt and freshly ground pepper and set aside.

2. Heat the oil in a large, wide frying pan over high heat to 370°F. Add the tortilla strips and fry until crisp and golden brown. This should only take a few seconds. Drain on paper towels.

3. Discard all but 2 tablespoons of the oil. Allow to cool for a few minutes. Reduce heat to low. Add the onions and peppers and sauté until the onions are soft but not brown. Add tomatoes and cook very briefly, about 1 minute. Season with a little sea salt, and transfer to a bowl.

4. Melt the butter in the frying pan and add the eggs. Cook slowly over low heat, stirring. When the eggs are somewhat set, stir in the vegetables. Just before the eggs are set, stir in the fried tortilla strips. Stir in the chopped, fresh coriander and serve at once.

12 eggs
Sea salt and freshly ground black pepper to taste
½ cup safflower or vegetable oil
6 corn tortillas (may be stale), cut into strips
½ small onion, minced
4 fresh or canned jalapeño or serrano peppers, seeded and chopped
4 medium-sized tomatoes, seeded and chopped
2 tablespoons butter
1 tablespoon chopped fresh coriander

Hard-Boiled Eggs and Tomatoes with Spices

Serves 4

4 hard-boiled eggs, shelled, cut in half
4 large ripe tomatoes, cut in wedges
½ teaspoon each sea salt, garam masala (see page 27), ground coriander, ground cumin
Freshly ground pepper
Chopped fresh parsley, chives, or coriander for garnish

Arrange the eggs and tomatoes on a platter. Mix together the sea salt and spices and sprinkle over the eggs and tomatoes. Add a little freshly ground pepper and garnish with fresh parsley, chives, or coriander. Serve as an hors d'oeuvre, as a first course, or as part of a light meal with other salads.

Curried Deviled Eggs

Serves 4

4 large eggs, hard-boiled
curry mayonnaise (page 155), to taste
Dijon style mustard to taste
Sweet paprika

Peel the eggs and cut in half. Gently remove the yolks and mash. Moisten to taste with curry mayonnaise and Dijon-style mustard. Gently spoon or pipe back into the whites. Sprinkle with paprika and arrange on a platter. Serve chilled or at room temperature as an hors d'oeuvre.

Spiced Tomato Buttermilk

This can be eaten as a cold soup or used as a sauce for rice.

Makes 2½ cups

1 tablespoon safflower or vegetable oil
4 cloves garlic, peeled and thinly sliced
½ hot green chili pepper, minced
¼ teaspoon cumin seeds
1 large ripe tomato, peeled, seeded and chopped
¾ cup water
Sea salt to taste
1 cup buttermilk
1 tablespoon chopped fresh coriander

1. Heat the oil in a frying pan and gently sauté the garlic until golden. Add the chili pepper and cumin, and sauté another couple of seconds. Add the tomato and water, stir together, and simmer 10 minutes. Remove from the heat and allow to cool.

2. Stir in the tomato mixture into the buttermilk. Add sea salt to taste and stir in the chopped fresh coriander. Serve over grains or as a cold soup.

ROASTED EGGPLANT RAITA

This is adapted from a recipe by Madhur Jaffrey.

2 green onions
¾ pound eggplant
2 cups plain low-fat yogurt
1 clove garlic, minced or put through a press
¾ teaspoon ground cumin
½ teaspoon paprika
3 tablespoons chopped fresh mint (optional)
Sea salt and freshly ground pepper to taste
Fresh lemon juice to taste (optional)

1. Slice the onions and set aside.

2. Preheat the oven to 450°F. Cut the eggplant in half lengthwise and score down to the skin but not through it, down the middle of the eggplant. Place on an oiled baking sheet cut side down and bake in the preheated oven until thoroughly soft on the inside and charred on the outside, or about 30 minutes. Remove from the heat and allow to cool. Scrape out the flesh when cool enough to handle, and discard the skin. Dice very small or mash.

3. Beat the yogurt with a whisk or fork until smooth. Stir in the eggplant and remaining ingredients. Season to taste with sea salt, chopped fresh mint, pepper, and lemon juice. Chill or serve at room temperature.

Spicy Banana Raita

Makes 2 cups

Beat the yogurt with a whisk or fork until smooth. Stir in the remaining ingredients. Correct seasonings. Serve on the side with vegetable curries or over grains.

1 cup plain low-fat yogurt
½ to 1 fresh hot green chili, to taste, minced
1 teaspoon mild-flavored honey
1 firm, ripe banana, diced
Sea salt and freshly ground pepper to taste

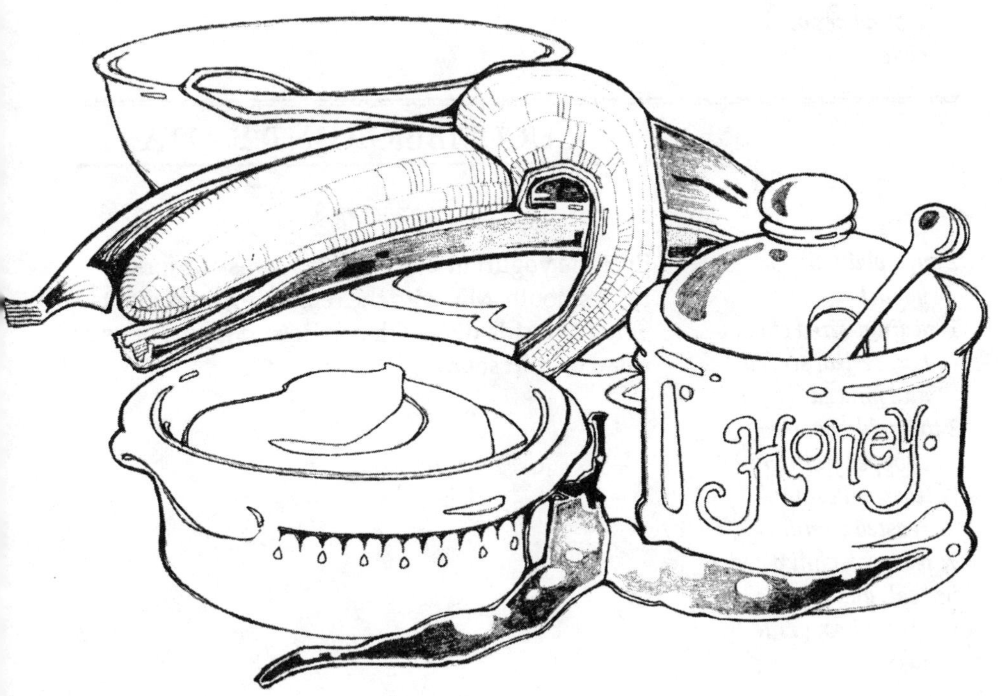

Spicy Cucumber Raita

This is adapted from a recipe by Madhur Jaffrey.

Makes 2 cups; serves 4

1 cup plain low-fat yogurt
⅛ teaspoon cayenne
2 tablespoons chopped fresh coriander
1 teaspoon black mustard seeds, crushed
1 medium-sized cucumber, peeled and grated
Sea salt and freshly ground pepper to taste

Beat the yogurt until smooth with a whisk or fork. Add the remaining ingredients. Chill and serve with grains or vegetable curries.

Cucumber-Mint Raita

Serves 6

2 cups plain low-fat yogurt
1 medium-sized cucumber, peeled, seeded, and minced
2 to 3 tablespoons chopped fresh mint
¾ teaspoon ground roasted cumin
¼ teaspoon chili powder
Sea salt and freshly ground pepper to taste

Beat the yogurt in a bowl with a whisk or fork until smooth. Mix with the remaining ingredients. Serve as a side dish with curries and grains or as a salad or cold soup.

Corn Pudding

Serves 4

1 tablespoon butter
1 small onion, minced
1 green pepper, chopped
1 teaspoon crushed cumin seeds
¼ teaspoon chili powder
1 canned or fresh jalapeño, seeded and chopped
2 cups fresh corn kernels, coarsely puréed
½ cup milk
4 eggs
½ teaspoon sweet paprika
Sea salt and freshly ground pepper to taste

1. Preheat the oven to 375°F. Butter a 2-quart soufflé dish.

2. Heat the butter in a heavy-bottomed frying pan and sauté the onion and green pepper until the onion is tender, or about 3 minutes. Add the cumin seeds, chili powder, jalapeño, and corn kernels, and continue to sauté, stirring, for another 3 minutes. Remove from the heat.

3. Separate 2 of the eggs. Beat together the whole eggs, egg yolks, and milk. Add the corn mixture, paprika, and salt and freshly ground pepper to taste.

4. Beat the egg whites until they form stiff peaks and fold into the corn mixture. Carefully turn into the buttered soufflé dish and bake for 30 minutes, or until the top is browned and the mixture set.

LEEK AND POTATO QUICHE WITH CUMIN

Serves 6

For the Crust:

1 cup whole wheat pastry flour
½ cup unbleached white flour
½ cup wheat germ
½ teaspoon sea salt
6 ounces cold unsalted butter
2 to 3 tablespoons ice-cold water

For the Filling:

1 tablespoon butter
2 leeks, white part only, cleaned and thinly sliced
¾ pound new potatoes, diced
1 teaspoon crushed cumin seeds
¼ teaspoon paprika
3 large eggs, at room temperature
1 cup milk
2 tablespoons dried milk
¼ teaspoon sea salt
Pinch of freshly grated nutmeg
Freshly ground pepper to taste
4 ounces Gruyère cheese, grated
2 ounces Parmesan cheese, grated
Freshly ground pepper

1. First make the pie crust. Mix together the flours, wheat germ, and sea salt, and cut in the butter. Add the water and gather into a ball. Wrap in plastic wrap and chill at least 1 hour or prefer-ably overnight. Roll out and line a 12-inch quiche pan. Pinch an attractive lip around the edge. Trim excess pastry and save for another purpose.

2. Preheat the oven to 350°F. Prick the pastry in several places with a fork and prebake 5 minutes. Remove from the heat.

3. Steam the potatoes until tender, about 10 minutes, and set aside.

4. Heat the butter in a frying pan and add the leeks. Sauté until they begin to soften and add the cumin, potatoes, and paprika. Continue to sauté another 5 minutes and remove from the heat.

5. Blend together the eggs, milk, dry milk, nutmeg, and freshly ground pepper in a blender.

6. Toss the cheeses together with the leeks and potatoes. Line the prebaked crust with this mixture. Place in the oven and bake 30 to 40 minutes, or until firm to the touch and begin-ning to brown on top. Remove from the heat, let sit about 5 minutes, and serve.

Spiced Cottage Cheese

Makes 1½ cups

Blend together the cottage cheese and yogurt. Stir in the remaining ingredients. Correct seasonings. Use as a sandwich spread (especially good on dark sour bread) or as a dip for vegetables.

1 cup cottage cheese
⅓ cup plain low-fat yogurt
1¼ teaspoons garam masala (see page 27)
⅛ teaspoon cayenne
2 teaspoons lemon juice, or to taste

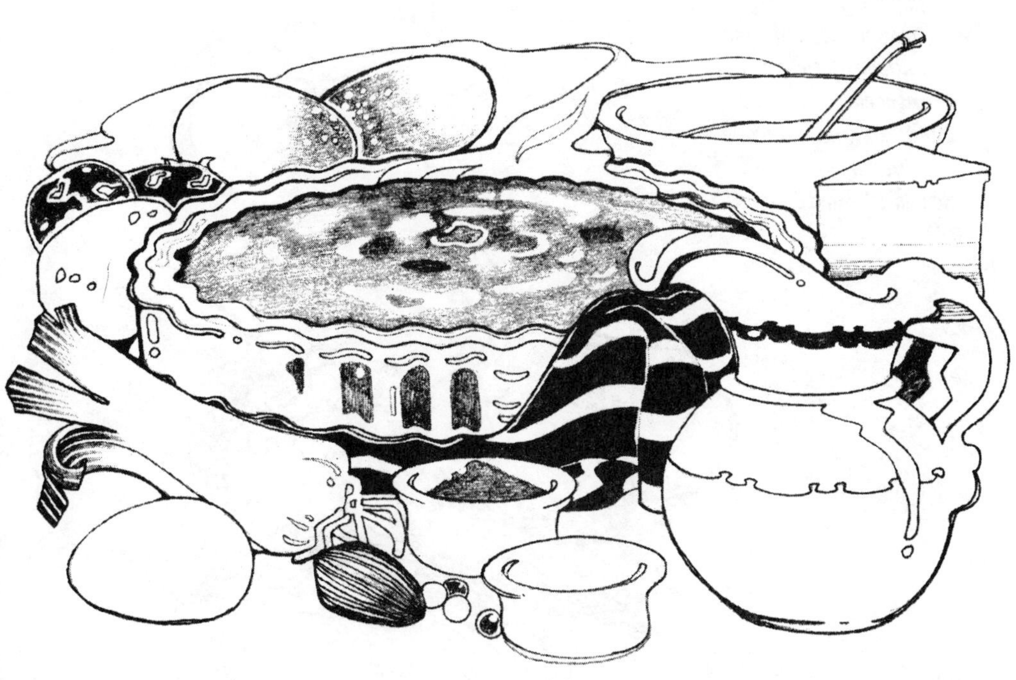

6
MEXICAN AND TEX-MEX DISHES

Salsa Fresca

Makes about 1½ cups

1 pound ripe tomatoes, chopped
½ small onion, minced
3 tablespoons chopped fresh coriander
2 serrano or jalapeño peppers, fresh or canned, seeded (use rubber gloves) and minced
2 tablespoons red wine vinegar
Sea salt to taste

Mix together all the ingredients in a bowl and serve, or chill and serve. This will hold for a day or two.

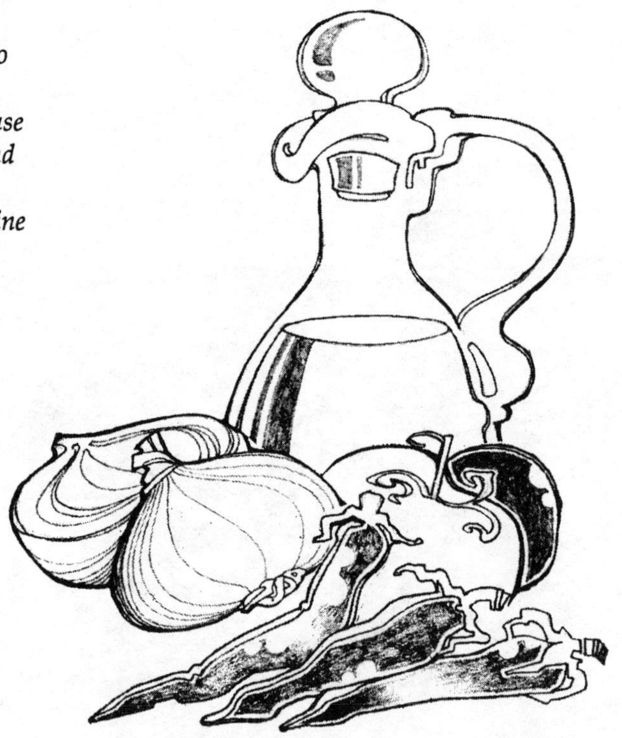

Green Tomato Sauce

Makes 2 cups

1. Remove the papery husks from the green tomatoes and place the tomatoes in a saucepan. Cover with water and bring to a simmer. Simmer gently for 10 minutes, or until soft.
2. Meanwhile, if using fresh serrano peppers, roast the peppers over a flame or in a dry skillet until they blister. When cool enough to handle, remove the stems (remove the stems of canned peppers if using).
3. When the tomatoes are soft, drain and blend them to a purée, along with the hot peppers, in a blender.
4. Heat the oil in a frying pan and add the minced onion and garlic. Sauté until the onion is tender and add the green tomato purée. Sauté over medium heat for 5 minutes, then remove from the heat. Serve hot or cold, or as a topping for enchiladas or tacos.

1 pound green Mexican tomatoes, available in Mexican groceries and some produce markets and supermarkets
2 fresh serrano peppers or canned jalapeños
2 cloves garlic, minced or put through a press
½ medium onion, minced
1 tablespoon safflower or vegetable oil
Sea salt to taste

Mexican-Style Beans

Serves 4 to 6

1 pound pinto beans, washed, picked over, and soaked
1 onion, chopped
4 cloves garlic, minced or put through a press
1 tablespoon safflower or vegetable oil
6 cups water
1 to 2 canned or fresh jalapeño peppers, to taste, cut in half, seeds and membranes removed
2 sprigs epazote, if available
1 teaspoon ground cumin
Sea salt to taste
4 to 5 tablespoons fresh chopped coriander

1. Soak the beans overnight and drain.

2. Heat the oil in a large, heavy-bottomed bean pot or casserole and sauté the onion with half the garlic until tender. Add the beans, water, peppers, epazote, and cumin. Bring to a boil, cover, reduce heat, and simmer 1 hour.

3. Add the sea salt, coriander, and remaining garlic, and continue to simmer another hour, or until the beans are tender and the broth aromatic. Serve with fresh corn tortillas, rice, or cornbread.

Note: These freeze well and will keep for 2 to 3 days in the refrigerator.

Refried Beans

Serves 4 to 6

1 pound pinto or black beans, washed, picked over, and soaked overnight
1 onion, chopped
4 cloves garlic, minced or put through a press
1 tablespoon safflower or vegetable oil
6 cups water
Sea salt to taste
4 tablespoons chopped fresh coriander
2–3 tablespoons additional safflower or vegetable oil
1 tablespoon ground chili powder
1 tablespoon ground cumin

1. First cook the beans. Heat 1 tablespoon of oil in a large, heavy-bottomed soup pot or casserole and sauté the onion and half the garlic until tender. Drain the beans and add along with the water. Bring to a boil, reduce heat, cover, and simmer 1 hour.

2. Add sea salt to taste and the remaining garlic and coriander, and simmer another hour, or until tender.

3. Drain the beans and retain about half the cooking liquid. Purée ⅔ of the beans in a food processor or blender, not until smooth but leaving some texture. Use some of the cooking liquid to moisten. You can also mash the beans with the back of a spoon or with a potato masher as you fry them.

4. Heat 1 tablespoon of the oil in a large, heavy-bottomed frying pan (nonstick is good here) and add half the cumin and chili powder. Sauté a minute, then add half the puréed beans and half the whole beans. Sauté, stirring and mashing with the back of your spoon, for about 15 or 20 minutes or longer, adding a little cooking liquid if they seem too dry. They should bubble while a crust forms on the bottom and they develop a kind of toasty aroma. Transfer to an ovenproof casserole and repeat this step with the remaining ingredients. Correct seasonings and keep warm in a low oven.

Note: These freeze well and will keep for 2 to 3 days in the refrigerator.

Bean Burritos

Serves 6

6 whole wheat flour tortillas (available in natural food stores)
2 cups cooked Mexican-style beans (page 140)
1 teaspoon ground cumin
1 teaspoon chili powder
1 tablespoon safflower, corn, or vegetable oil
2 ounces grated cheddar or Monterey jack cheese
1 cup shredded lettuce or alfalfa sprouts
2 to 3 tomatoes, chopped

1. Preheat the oven to 325°F. Wrap the tortillas in foil and place in the oven while you prepare the beans.

2. Drain the beans, retaining about ½ cup of their liquid. Coarsely purée, using the pulse action, in a food processor or blender, along with the cumin and chili powder. Moisten with the bean broth.

3. Heat the oil in a large frying pan and add the beans. Sauté, stirring, about 10 minutes.

4. Remove the tortillas from the oven and spread the refried beans down the center. Top with the cheese and roll up. Heat in the oven for about 15 to 20 minutes, or until the cheese melts. Serve with the chopped tomatoes and lettuce on the side.

Meatless Chili

Serves 4 to 6

2 onions, chopped
4 large cloves garlic, minced or put through a press
1 tablespoon safflower oil
2 large carrots, chopped or grated
1 large bell pepper, chopped
2 large cans tomatoes, drained and chopped, or 3 pounds fresh ripe tomatoes, chopped
1 small can tomato paste
1 bay leaf
1 tablespoon chili powder
2 teaspoons cumin
2 dried cayenne peppers, or ¼ teaspoon cayenne pepper
1 or 2 dried poblano chilies, if available (optional)
Sea salt and freshly ground pepper to taste
1 pound red or kidney beans, cooked (may use canned)
½ cup of the liquid from the beans
1 teaspoon oregano

1. Heat the safflower oil in a large, heavy-bottomed casserole or soup pot. Add the onions and half the garlic and sauté until the onion begins to soften. Add the carrots and pepper and continue to sauté another 3 to 5 minutes, stirring all the while with a wooden spoon.

2. Add the tomatoes, tomato paste, bay leaf, and spice, and bring to a simmer. Crumble in the optional dried poblano pepper and add the remaining garlic. Reduce heat, cover, and simmer over very low heat, stirring occasionally, for 30 minutes. Stir in the beans and their liquid and the oregano, and continue to cook another 30 minutes. Check from time to time and stir to be sure that the chili doesn't stick. Adjust seasonings, adding salt, pepper, garlic, or cayenne to taste.

3. Serve with cornbread or corn tortillas or with whole wheat bread and a big green salad.

Spiced Nacho Chips

The nacho chips you make at home will taste much better than the ones that come out of a bag. You need a tortilla press and a heavy cast iron skillet or, even better, a comal *or a Mexican griddle, for these. Masa harina is a special kind of cornmeal for corn tortilla.*

Makes 24 chips

2 cloves garlic, peeled and sliced very thin
1 tablespoon safflower or vegetable oil
2 cups masa harina
¼ cup unbleached white flour
½ teaspoon sea salt
½ teaspoon ground cumin
½ teaspoon chili powder
1 cup plus 2 to 3 tablespoons water, as needed
2 plastic bags
1 quart safflower, vegetable, or corn oil for deep-frying

1. Heat 1 tablespoon of oil and sauté the sliced garlic for 2 minutes, stirring. Set aside.

2. Mix together the masa harina, flour, sea salt, cumin, and chili powder in a bowl. Stir in the sautéed garlic. Pour in 1 cup of the water all at once and mix together quickly with your hands. Dough should not be in a big lump but should be slightly crumbly and not too dry. If the dough seems too dry, add a little water, a tablespoon at a time. Let rest for 15 minutes.

3. Take up small marble-sized pieces of the dough and shape into little balls.

4. Heat a *comal* griddle or heavy-bottomed frying pan over medium-high heat. To press out the tortilla chips place one of the plastic bags on your tortilla press and one, two, or three balls, widely spaced, on top of this. Press down a little with your thumb, and place the other plastic bag on top. Now press the tortillas, being careful not to press too hard or your tortilla chips will be too thin. Lift the press and peel off the top bag. Flip the tortillas gently onto the peeled-off bag and peel off the bottom bag.

5. Transfer the little tortillas to the hot *comal* or frying pan and cook about 1 minute, or until the tortillas are just beginning to dry around the edges. Turn and cook another minute. Remove from the heat.

6. To make the final chips, heat the oil to 370°F. in a deep frying pan, saucepan, or wok and add the chips, a few at a time. Deep-fry until crisp and golden. This should only take a few seconds. Drain on paper towels and toss with sea salt to taste.

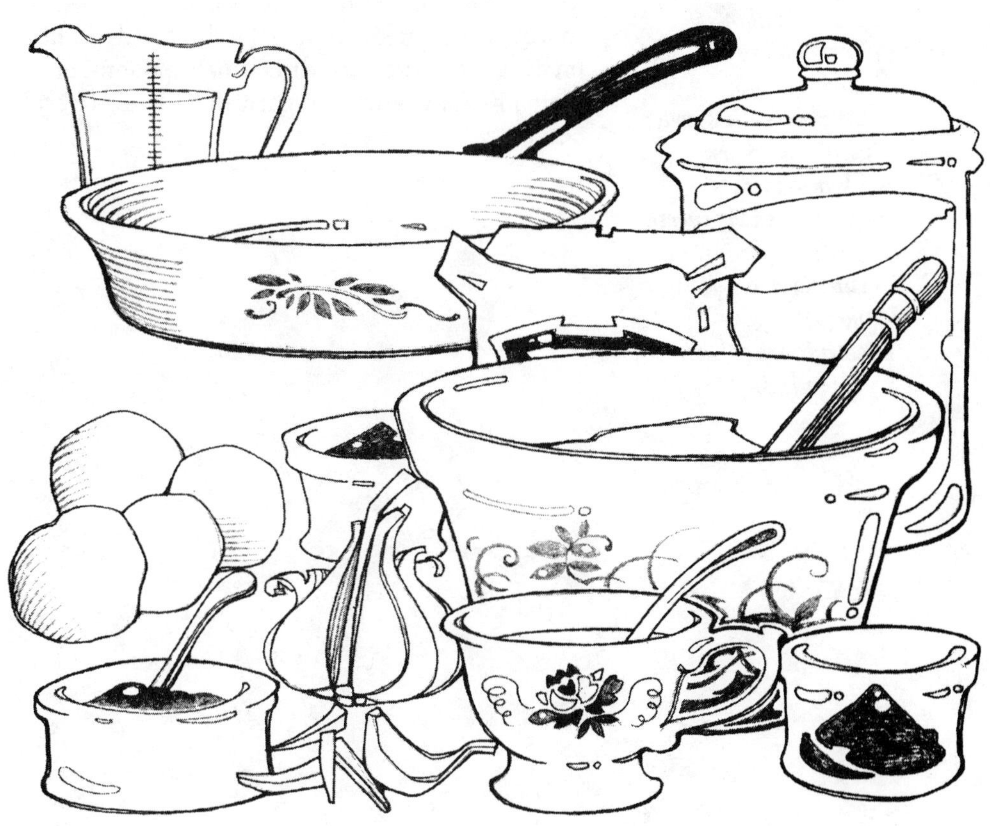

Guacamole Nachos

Makes 24 to 30 nachos

8 corn tortillas
Oil for deep-frying
2 ripe avocados
1 small ripe tomato, chopped
1 small clove garlic, minced or put through a press
1 tablespoon finely minced onion
¼ teaspoon ground cumin
¼ teaspoon chili powder
Juice of 1 large lemon
Sea salt to taste
2 ounces cheddar cheese, grated
⅓ cup plain low-fat yogurt
4 tablespoons salsa fresca (page 138)

1. Cut the tortillas into quarters. Heat the oil to 360°F. and deep-fry until crisp and golden. This should only take a few seconds. Drain on paper towels.

2. Mash together the avocados, tomato, garlic, and onion. Season with the cumin, chili powder, lemon juice, and sea salt to taste.

3. Heat the broiler. Sprinkle the grated cheese over the chips and melt under the broiler. When thoroughly melted, remove the chips and spoon on the guacamole, top with a small spoonful of plain low-fat yogurt, and garnish with salsa fresca. Serve.

Bean Nachos

Makes 24 nachos

6 corn tortillas
Safflower or vegetable oil for deep-frying
1 cup refried beans (page 141)
2 ounces cheddar or Monterey jack cheese, grated
4 canned jalapeño chilies, cut in rounds

1. Cut the corn tortillas into quarters. Heat the safflower oil to 360°F. and deep-fry the tortillas until golden and crisp. This should only take a few seconds. Drain on paper towels.

2. Preheat the broiler. Place 2 heaped teaspoons of the refried beans on each nacho chip. Sprinkle the cheese over the beans and broil briefly to melt the cheese. Garnish with a round of jalapeño pepper and serve.

Bean and Avocado Chalupas

Serves 4 to 6

1 recipe refried beans (page 141)
2 large or 3 small, ripe avocados, preferably the dark, knobby Haas variety
1 small serrano pepper, minced
4 tomatoes, chopped
Juice of 1 lemon
1 small onion, minced
1 small clove garlic, minced or put through a press
½ teaspoon ground cumin
½ teaspoon chili powder
Sea salt to taste
1 tablespoon red wine vinegar
1 to 2 additional serrano or jalapeño peppers, chopped
3 to 4 tablespoons chopped fresh coriander
6 ounces cheddar cheese, grated
1½ cups shredded lettuce
8 to 12 flat corn tortilla chips (chalupa chips)
(You can deep-fry your own corn tortillas if you can't find tortilla chips.)

1. Make the refried beans and set aside (keep warm in a medium oven if you are serving the chalupas soon).

2. Mash the avocados together with one of the tomatoes, one chopped serrano pepper, a quarter of the onions (more to taste), the garlic, cumin, chili powder, lemon juice, and sea salt to taste. Correct seasonings, adding more lemon juice or spices if you wish.

3. Chop the remaining 3 tomatoes and toss with the remaining onion, vinegar, chopped serranos or jalapeño, chopped fresh coriander, and sea salt to taste.

4. Have all the ingredients in separate bowls. To assemble the chalupas, spread a generous spoonful of refried beans on each tortilla crisp, and top with the avocado purée, then some grated cheese, shredded lettuce, and the tomato salsa.

Stuffed Jalapeños

Serves 4 to 6

6 canned pickled jalapeño peppers
¼ pound ricotta cheese
¼ pound goat's cheese
¼ teaspoon ground cumin
Chopped fresh coriander as garnish

1. Wear rubber gloves, as the peppers will irritate your hands. Cut the jalapeños in half and discard the seeds.

2. Mash the two cheeses together in a bowl and stir in the cumin. Put the mixture into a pastry bag and pipe it into the jalapeño shells (or fill them with a spoon). Arrange on a plate and garnish with the coriander.

Mole Sauce

This is a rich Mexican sauce made with several kinds of dried chili peppers, spices, nuts, raisins, and even a little bit of chocolate. If you've never eaten mole (pronounced "molay") this recipe may look strange; but if you like complex, richly seasoned food, you will love it. It is fairly time-consuming, but it's worth the effort. No spice cookbook would be complete without this recipe. My vegetarian version is quite different from the authentic mole, which is made with a fearful amount of lard and calls for turkey stock rather than vegetable stock. But the richness of the spices comes through here, and that's the important thing. Mole is usually served with turkey or chicken. I serve it with cheese enchiladas *(see recipe, page 153)**; with hot, cooked grains; as a dip for raw vegetables; and even as a spread.*

Note: If you can't get the chili peppers listed here, use a different combination of those chilies you can get. The flavor will be slightly different, but it will still be mole.

Makes about 1 quart

8 dried chilies mulatos
5 dried chilies anchos
6 dried chilies pasillas
4 tablespoons safflower, corn, or vegetable oil
1 cup water
2 additional tablespoons safflower, corn, or vegetable oil
10 peppercorns
¼ teaspoon toasted cumin seeds
¼ teaspoon toasted coriander seeds
½ teaspoon cinnamon, or ½-inch stick

1. *The day before:* Split open the chilies and remove the seeds and membranes, retaining 1 tablespoon of the seeds for future use. Heat the first 4 tablespoons of the oil and sauté the chilies for about 2 minutes, being very careful not to burn them. Remove from the heat, place in a bowl, and cover with warm water. Soak overnight (you can toast the chili seeds and the spices during this time).

2. Drain the chilies and purée in a blender with 1 cup of water. Heat the next 2 tablespoons of oil in a large, heavy-bottomed frying pan and sauté the chili paste, stirring over medium-high heat, for 10 minutes. The mixture will sputter and you should use a lid to protect yourself. Set aside.

3. Grind together all the spices, along with the toasted chili seeds, in a spice mill. Transfer to a blender along with the tomato, garlic, and sesame seeds (a blender works better than a food processor here for achieving the correct texture).

4. Heat the remaining tablespoon of oil and sauté the raisins just until they plump. Transfer, using a slotted spoon, to the blender jar. Brown the almonds and the stale tortilla in the same oil (add more if necessary) and transfer to the blender jar. Add the bread. Now blend this mixture to a smooth paste, adding a little vegetable stock if necessary. Add this mixture to the chili paste and stir together well.

5. Sauté the chili mixture over medium heat for 5 minutes, stirring all the while. Add a little more oil if the mole sticks to the pan. Break the chocolate into small pieces and stir into the mixture. Continue to sauté, stirring occasionally, for 10 more minutes.

6. Now stir in the vegetable stock or bouillon and continue to cook, stirring from time to time, for about 40 minutes or longer if necessary. If the mixture seems too thick, add a little stock or water. If it is sputtering too much, partially cover with a lid. It should be thick and should coat both sides of a wooden spoon, but liquid enough to call a sauce. Add sea salt to taste and remove from the heat. This will hold for 2 to 3 days in the refrigerator and can be frozen.

1 tablespoon reserved chili seeds, toasted

4 tablespoons sesame seeds, toasted

1 large ripe tomato, peeled

3 cloves garlic, toasted in a dry frying pan until brown and set aside

1 additional tablespoon safflower, corn, or vegetable oil

2 tablespoons raisins

30 almonds

4 pieces toasted or stale French or whole wheat bread

1 stale corn tortilla

1½ ounces Mexican or bitter chocolate

4 to 5 cups vegetable stock or bouillon (pages 54 and 55)

Sea salt to taste

Green Rice with Stuffed Chilies

Serves 6

1 cup parsley
1/4 cup fresh coriander leaves
1/3 cup water
1/2 small onion, minced
2 cloves garlic, minced or put through a press
2 tablespoons safflower or vegetable oil
1 1/4 cups brown rice, preferably long grained, washed
3 cups water or vegetable stock (page 54)
1 cup milk
1/2 to 1 teaspoon sea salt, to taste
12 canned jalapeños, drained
3/4 pound mild cheddar cheese, grated
1/2 to 1 teaspoon ground cumin, to taste

1. Blend together the parsley, coriander leaves, and water in a blender. Set aside.

2. Heat the oil in a large, heavy-bottomed, lidded frying pan or casserole and add the onion and garlic. Sauté over medium heat until the onion is tender. Add the rice and sauté, stirring about 5 minutes. Stir in the blended parsley and coriander, and combine well.

3. Add the water or stock and milk and bring to a boil. Add the sea salt, cover, reduce heat, and simmer for 40 minutes while you prepare the chilies.

4. Cut the chilies down one side and carefully remove the seeds (wear rubber gloves to avoid irritating skin). Toss the grated cheese with the cumin. Stuff the chilies with the cheese. Bring the slit edges of the chilies as close together as you can.

5. Now set the chilies in the rice, slit side up. The rice should have been cooking for about 20 minutes at this point. Cook for another 20 minutes, covered, or until the rice is cooked al dente and all the liquid absorbed.

Cheese Enchiladas with Mole Sauce

Serves 6

18 corn tortillas
3 to 4 tablespoons safflower, corn, or vegetable oil
½ teaspoon chili powder
½ teaspoon ground cumin
Sea salt to taste
1 small can tomato sauce
¾ pound mild cheddar or Monterey jack cheese
1 small onion, minced
1 recipe mole sauce (page 150)
3 tablespoons toasted sesame seeds

1. Preheat the oven to 350°F. Oil a 2-quart baking dish.

2. Heat 2 tablespoons of the oil in a large, heavy-bottomed frying pan. Combine the spices and sea salt and add a generous pinch to the oil. Add 2 to 3 tablespoons of tomato sauce and stir together. Sauté the tortillas on each side, just until flexible, being careful not to crisp, and drain on paper towels.

3. Sprinkle 2 to 3 tablespoons of cheese and a smattering of onion on each tortilla and roll up. Place in a neat line in the baking dish (you may have to do two layers). Cover with foil and place in the preheated oven. Bake 30 minutes, or until the cheese is bubbling.

4. Meanwhile heat the mole sauce on the top of the stove. If the sauce is too thick, thin out with water or vegetable stock. When the enchiladas are ready, spoon the sauce over the enchiladas, sprinkle with sesame seeds, and serve at once. You can also arrange two to three enchiladas on individual plates, top with the sauce, sprinkle with sesame seeds, and serve.

Potato and Avocado Tacos with Green Salsa

Makes 12 tacos

1 pound new or boiling potatoes, diced
3 to 4 tablespoons safflower oil
1 small onion, thinly sliced
½ teaspoon ground cumin
½ teaspoon chili powder
2 ripe avocados, diced and tossed with 1 tablespoon lemon juice
Sea salt to taste
¼ pound mild cheddar or Monterey jack cheese, grated
12 corn tortillas
1 recipe green tomato sauce (page 139)

1. Steam the potatoes until crisp-tender, about 10 minutes.

2. Heat 1 tablespoon of the safflower oil in a heavy-bottomed frying pan and sauté the onion until tender. Add cumin, chili powder, and the potatoes, and continue to sauté until the vegetables are just beginning to brown, about 10 minutes. Add more oil if necessary.

3. Remove the onions and potatoes from the heat and toss with the avocados. Add sea salt to taste.

4. Heat the tortillas until flexible in a dry frying pan. Place 2 heaped tablespoons of the potato-avocado mixture on each tortilla and top with a spoonful of green salsa and a sprinkling of grated cheese. Roll up like an enchilada, or fold in half.

5. Heat the remaining oil in the frying pan and sauté the tacos on both or all sides (depending on whether they are rolled or folded) just until crisp. Serve at once, topping each taco with additional green salsa.

7
SALADS AND DRESSINGS

CURRY MAYONNAISE

Makes 1¼ cups

1. Put everything except the oil and lemon juice in the bowl of a food processor or blender jar. Turn on and blend for a few seconds.

2. With the food processor or blender still running, add the oil in a very slow stream, practically a drop at a time. If you are using a blender, you may have to stop and stir the mixture from time to time. When all the oil has been added, add the lemon juice. Taste and adjust seasonings, adding salt, lemon juice, or curry powder to taste. If you want the mayonnaise slightly sweet, add up to 1 teaspoon honey.

1 egg
2 teaspoons red wine or cider vinegar
½ to ¾ teaspoon sea salt, to taste
1 teaspoon Dijon mustard
¼ teaspoon freshly ground pepper
2 teaspoons curry powder
¼ teaspoon chili powder
¼ teaspoon turmeric
1 cup safflower or vegetable oil
2 tablespoons lemon juice, or to taste
Up to 1 teaspoon mild-flavored honey (optional)

Curried Yogurt Dressing

Makes 1½ cups

Juice of 2 lemons
1 cup plain low-fat yogurt
3 tablespoons mayonnaise
1 teaspoon Dijon-style mustard
½ teaspoon turmeric
½ teaspoon chili powder
½ teaspoon freshly grated ginger
½ teaspoon paprika
2 teaspoons curry powder
Pinch of cayenne
Sea salt and freshly ground pepper to taste

Blend all the ingredients together and refrigerate until ready to use.

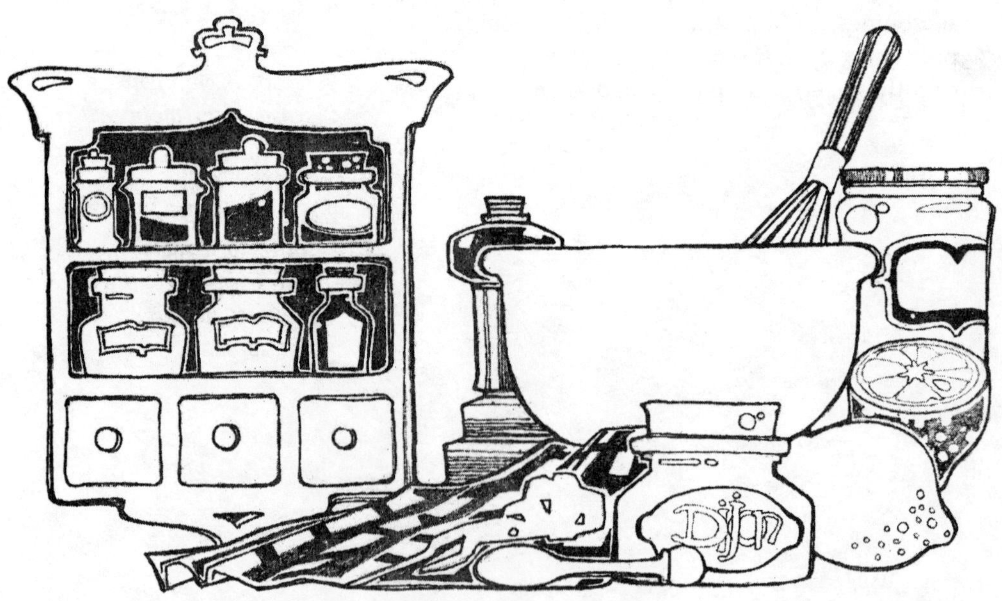

Lemon-Curry Vinaigrette

Makes ¾ cup

Combine the lemon juice, mustard, cumin, curry powder, sea salt, and soy sauce, and stir together well. Whisk in the oil and blend thoroughly. Add lots of freshly ground pepper.

¼ cup lemon juice
1 teaspoon Dijon mustard
½ teaspoon cumin
¼ teaspoon curry powder
Pinch of sea salt
¼ teaspoon soy sauce
½ cup safflower oil
A generous amount of freshly ground pepper

Honey-Lemon Salad Dressing

Makes ¾ cup

Combine the lemon juice, honey, mustard, pepper, ginger, and soy sauce and stir together well. Whisk in the oil and blend thoroughly.

¼ cup lemon juice
1 tablespoon mild-flavored honey
1 teaspoon Dijon mustard
Freshly ground pepper to taste
¼ teaspoon ground ginger, or ½ to ¾ teaspoon grated fresh ginger, to taste
¼ teaspoon soy sauce
½ cup safflower oil

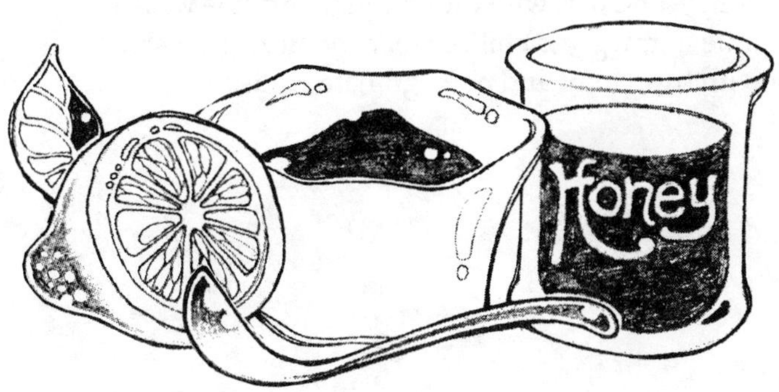

Moroccan Carrot Salad

Serves 4 to 6

1 pound carrots, peeled and grated
¾ cup minced fresh parsley
Pinch of sea salt
1 tablespoon orange flower water
1½ teaspoons mild-flavored honey
Juice of 2 lemons
¼ teaspoon allspice
½ teaspoon ground cumin
Leaf lettuce for the platter or bowl

1. Combine the carrots, parsley, and sea salt.
2. Stir together the orange flower water, honey, lemon juice, allspice, and cumin. Just before serving toss with the carrots.
3. Line a platter or bowl with lettuce leaves, top with the carrots, and serve.

Moroccan Orange Salad

Serves 4

1 tablespoon orange flower water
⅛ to ¼ teaspoon cinnamon, to taste
1 teaspoon mild-flavored honey
6 oranges, peels and zest removed, cut in thin slices
Pinch of nutmeg
Fresh chopped mint for garnish
Pomegranate seeds for garnish

Combine the orange flower water, cinnamon, and honey, and toss with the oranges. Sprinkle with a little nutmeg and chill, or serve at once, garnishing with fresh mint and pomegranate seeds.

Mexican Rice Salad

Serves 6 to 8

For the Salad:
1 cup brown rice
2 cups water
½ teaspoon saffron
Sea salt and freshly ground pepper to taste
½ pound green beans, trimmed and blanched
1 red pepper, seeded and cut in thin strips
4 green onions, chopped
4 to 5 tablespoons pine nuts, to taste
1 small cucumber, peeled, seeded and chopped
3 to 4 tablespoons chopped, fresh coriander, to taste

For the Dressing:
3 tablespoons wine or cider vinegar
Juice of 1 large lemon
1 clove garlic, minced or put through a press
1 teaspoon Dijon-style mustard
1 teaspoon ground cumin
½ cup safflower oil
¼ cup olive oil
Sea salt and freshly ground pepper to taste
Leaf lettuce for the bowl or platter (optional)

1. Cook the brown rice in the water with the saffron and sea salt to taste. Meanwhile, prepare the vegetables and the dressing.

2. To prepare the dressing, mix together the vinegar, lemon juice, garlic, mustard, and ground cumin. Blend in the oils and combine well. Add sea salt and freshly ground pepper to taste.

3. Allow the rice to cool, then toss with the vegetables and the dressing. Chill for an hour or two, adjust seasonings, and serve, lining bowl or platter, if you wish, with lettuce leaves.

Cold Minted Potatoes

Serves 6

2 pounds red waxy or new potatoes
2 medium-sized cucumbers, or 1 long cucumber, peeled, seeded, and diced
Sea salt to taste
Juice of 2 lemons
1 teaspoon ground roasted cumin (see page 7)
1 teaspoon ground roasted coriander (see page 7)
¼ teaspoon ground black pepper
Pinch of cayenne, or to taste
6 heaping tablespoons plain low-fat yogurt
¼ cup chopped fresh mint

1. Steam the potatoes until tender, about 20 minutes, and dice.

2. Toss the potatoes with the cucumber, sea salt, lemon juice, spices, yogurt, and mint. Chill for at least 1 hour, and serve.

Note: This will keep for 3 to 4 days in the refrigerator

Spicy Eggplant Salad

Serves 4

1. Cut the eggplant in strips about 2 inches long, ½ inch thick, and 1 inch wide. Steam 15 minutes, or until tender. Drain, rinse, and pat dry with paper towels.
2. Steam the snow peas for 5 minutes and refresh under cold water. Drain and set aside.
3. Combine the ingredients for the dressing and blend together well. Toss with the eggplant, onions, and peas. Refrigerate for 2 hours or more. Toss with the optional coriander just before serving.

For the Salad:

1 pound eggplant, peeled
½ pound snow peas, trimmed
4 green onions, sliced
1 tablespoon chopped fresh coriander

For the Dressing:

2 to 3 tablespoons cider or white wine vinegar (to taste)
1 clove garlic, minced or put through a press
1 teaspoon finely minced or grated fresh ginger
1 tablespoon tamari soy sauce
2 tablespoons water
½ teaspoon crushed dried hot pepper, or ⅛ to ¼ teaspoon cayenne, to taste
4 tablespoons safflower or vegetable oil
2 tablespoons sesame oil

Spicy Potato Salad with Coriander

Serves 6

2 pounds red waxy or new potatoes
1 pound ripe tomatoes, diced
4 green onions, minced
1 clove garlic, minced or put through a press
1 teaspoon ground roasted cumin (see page 6)
Juice of 1 to 2 lemons, to taste
Sea salt to taste
Freshly ground pepper to taste

1. Steam the potatoes until tender, about 20 minutes.

2. Drain, refresh under cold water, and toss with remaining ingredients. Chill at least 1 hour.

Note: This will keep 3 days in the refrigerator.

Indian Peach Salad

Serves 6

1 tablespoon honey
3 tablespoons lemon or lime juice
¼ teaspoon sea salt
Freshly ground pepper to taste
1½ teaspoons ground roasted cumin
⅛ teaspoon cayenne pepper
2 pounds fresh peaches, peeled and sliced

Mix together the honey, lemon or lime juice, salt, pepper, cumin, and cayenne. Toss this dressing with the peaches. Serve.

Millet-Lentil Salad

Serves 4 to 6

For the Dressing:
½ cup lemon juice
1 clove garlic, minced or put through a press
2 teaspoons curry powder
½ teaspoon ground cumin
¼ teaspoon ground coriander
1 teaspoon grated, fresh ginger
Pinch of cayenne
Sea salt and freshly ground pepper, to taste
1 cup plain low-fat yogurt

For the Salad:
1 cup millet, cooked
¾ cup lentils, washed and cooked
½ pound carrots, peeled and thinly sliced
4 to 6 green onions, thinly sliced
½ cup chopped fresh parsley
Lettuce leaves for garnish

1. Mix together all the ingredients for the salad dressing and blend well.

2. Toss together the millet, lentils, carrots, green onions, and parsley. Toss with the dressing, cover, and chill for an hour or two. Serve over lettuce leaves.

Curried Grain Salad

Serves 6 to 8

1 recipe curried yogurt dressing (page 156)
1 cup raw brown rice, cooked
1 cup raw wheat berries, cooked
½ cup raw garbanzos, cooked
¼ cup freshly grated Parmesan cheese
1 medium-sized cucumber, peeled and chopped
1 green pepper, chopped
¼ cup lightly toasted peanuts (unsalted)
¼ cup raisins
1 apple, chopped
¼ to ½ cup chopped fresh parsley

For the Garnish:
1 head leaf lettuce
2 tomatoes, cut in wedges

1. Toss all the ingredients together with the dressing and chill for an hour or so.

2. Line a bowl or platter with lettuce leaves and top with the salad. Garnish with the tomatoes and serve.

Endive, Apple, and Mushroom Salad

Serves 4

1. Toss together all the ingredients for the salad.
2. Mix together the ingredients for the dressing and blend well. Toss with the salad and serve.

For the Salad:

½ pound endive, sliced in 1-inch pieces
½ pound mushrooms, cleaned, trimmed, and thinly sliced
2 tart apples, cored and sliced
3 tablespoons chopped walnuts
1 tablespoon chopped fresh chives
3 tablespoons minced fresh parsley

For the Dressing:

Juice of 1 lemon
½ teaspoon Dijon mustard
½ teaspoon mild-flavored honey
½ cup plain low-fat yogurt
¾ teaspoon curry powder
¼ teaspoon ground cumin

Spicy Noodle Salad

Serves 6

For the Dressing:
2 tablespoons crunchy unsalted peanut butter
1 tablespoon soy sauce
3 tablespoons white wine or cider vinegar
1 tablespoon hot Chinese pepper oil (page 172)
2 tablespoons sesame oil
1 tablespoon minced fresh ginger
1 clove garlic, minced or put through a press
¾ cup Vegetable stock (page 54) or bouillon

For the Salad:
½ pound whole wheat or buckwheat noodles
2 tablespoons sesame oil
4 green onions, sliced thin
3 tablespoons chopped fresh coriander
Lettuce leaves for garnish

1. Blend together all the ingredients for the dressing in a blender until smooth.

2. Bring a large pot of water to a boil and add 1 teaspoon of sea salt and the noodles. Cook until al dente, 4 to 10 minutes, depending on the kind of noodle, drain, and refresh under cold water. Toss at once with the sesame oil, green onions, and coriander. Toss again with the dressing and correct seasonings, adding soy sauce, salt, pepper, or cayenne if you wish. Line a platter with lettuce leaves and top with the noodles. Chill and serve, or serve at once.

Note: The ginger-flavored buckwheat noodles on page 122 would be particularly good here.

Spiced Carrot Salad

Serves 4 to 6

2 pounds carrots, peeled and grated
3 tablespoons grated onion
Juice of 1 large lemon
1 teaspoon Dijon mustard
2 teaspoons curry powder
½ teaspoon ground cumin
½ teaspoon chili powder
¼ teaspoon ground allspice
Pinch of cayenne
Sea salt and freshly ground pepper to taste
¼ cup safflower oil
3 tablespoons plain low-fat yogurt
2 tablespoons chopped fresh coriander or parsley

1. Toss together the carrots and grated onion.

2. Mix together the lemon juice, mustard, spices, salt, pepper, safflower oil, and yogurt. Combine well and toss with the grated carrots. Correct seasonings, adding more spices if you wish. Sprinkle the chopped fresh coriander or parsley over the top and serve, or chill and serve.

Oriental Cucumber Salad

Serves 4

3 tablespoons white wine or cider vinegar
1 tablespoon soy sauce
2 teaspoons mild-flavored honey
1 small clove garlic, minced or put through a press
1 teaspoon minced fresh ginger
1/8 to 1/4 teaspoon cayenne or hot red pepper flakes
Freshly ground pepper to taste
2 tablespoons sesame oil
4 tablespoons safflower oil
2 large cucumbers, peeled and sliced thin
3 green onions, green part and white, sliced thin
2 tablespoons chopped fresh coriander

1. Mix together the vinegar, soy sauce, honey, garlic, ginger and cayenne. Add freshly ground pepper to taste and whisk in the sesame oil and safflower oil. Correct seasonings.

2. Toss together the cucumbers, onions, and coriander. Toss with the dressing and serve, or chill and serve.

Cauliflower and Fresh Pea Salad

Serves 4 to 6

1 pound cauliflower (about ½ head), broken into florets and sliced ½-inch thick
1 cup fresh peas
Juice of ½ to 1 lemon, to taste
2 cups plain low-fat yogurt
1 clove garlic, minced or put through a press
1 teaspoon Dijon mustard (optional)
½ teaspoon ground roasted cumin seeds (more to taste)
Sea salt and freshly ground pepper to taste
Cayenne pepper to taste
2 tablespoons chopped fresh coriander, mint, or chives (optional)

1. Steam the cauliflower and the peas separately until crisp-tender, about 5 minutes for the cauliflower and 10 minutes for the peas. Drain and refresh under cold water.

2. Mix together the lemon juice, yogurt, garlic, optional mustard, cumin, sea salt, pepper, and cayenne. Toss with the cauliflower and peas. Chill until ready to serve. Toss with the optional coriander, mint, or chives just before serving.

Watercress, Orange, Fennel, and Tomato Salad

Serves 4

2 cups watercress, trimmed, washed, and dried
1 bulb fennel, sliced very thin
2 oranges, peeled, white pith removed, sectioned
2 large ripe tomatoes, cut in thin wedges
1 tablespoon chopped fresh mint

For the Dressing:
Juice of 1 lemon
½ teaspoon freshly grated ginger
½ teaspoon Dijon mustard
¾ cup plain low-fat yogurt
1 teaspoon curry powder
¼ teaspoon ground cumin
Sea salt and freshly ground pepper to taste

1. Toss together the watercress, fennel, oranges, tomatoes, and mint.

2. Mix together the ingredients for the dressing and blend well. Toss with the salad just before serving.

8
SEASONINGS, DIPS, CHUTNEYS, AND BEVERAGES

North Indian Spice Mix

This tasty mixture, introduced to me by Madhur Jaffrey, makes a nice seasoning for raw vegetables and nuts.

2 tablespoons whole coriander seeds
1 tablespoon whole cumin
3 tablespoons sesame seeds
2 tablespoons coarse or regular sea salt
¼ teaspoon cayenne
¼ teaspoon black pepper

1. Roast the coriander seeds, cumin seeds, and sesame seeds. Allow to cool, then grind. Mix with the remaining ingredients.
2. Sprinkle on raw vegetables or on peanuts or other nuts or seeds such as sunflower seeds or pumpkin seeds, which have first been sprinkled with a little lime juice.

HOT CHINESE PEPPER OIL

Use this for spicy Szechuan or Hunan dishes. It will keep for months in the refrigerator.

½ cup safflower or vegetable oil
1½ teaspoons ground, hot, dried red peppers (such as cayenne)

1. Place the oil in a pan and heat until it begins to ripple. Add the ground, hot, dried red peppers and remove from the heat.

2. Allow to cool, then strain into a bottle. Store in the refrigerator. A teaspoon of this will add heat to any dish.

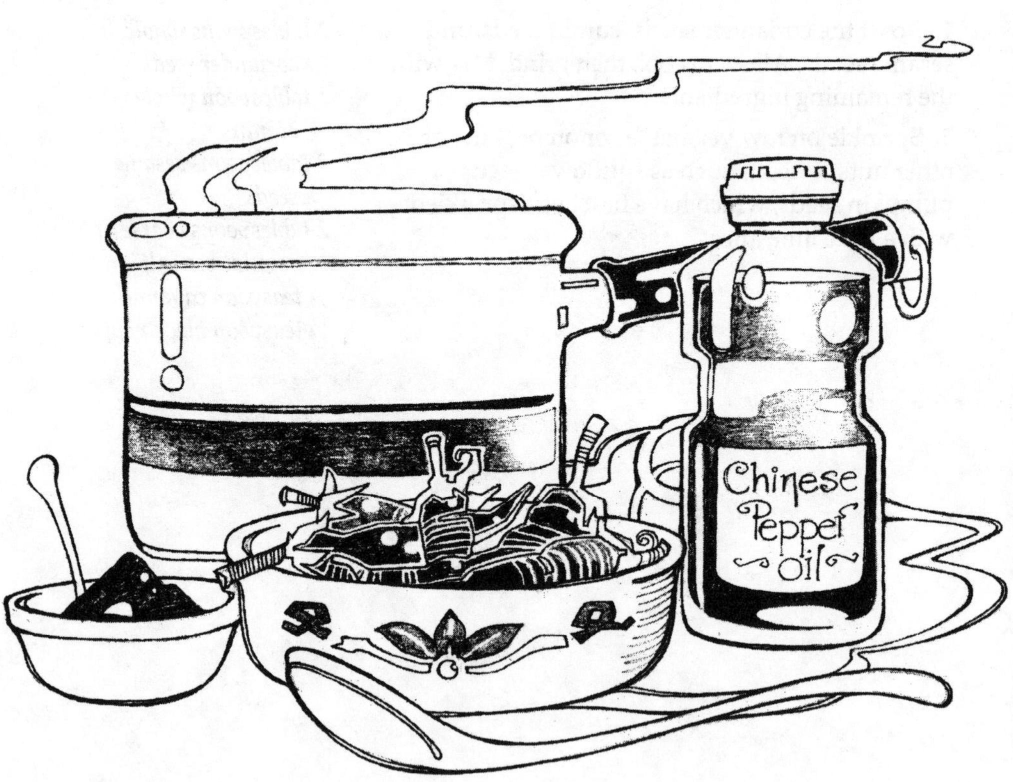

Pear-Apple Chutney

Makes 1 quart

1 pound apples, peeled, cored, and chopped
2 pounds pears, peeled, cored, and chopped
1 tablespoon peeled and minced fresh ginger
1 cup cider vinegar
½ cup mild-flavored honey
1 small onion, minced
3 cloves garlic, peeled and chopped
1 small hot green chili, seeded and minced
4 tablespoons raisins
1 teaspoon ground cardamom
½ teaspoon ground cloves
1 tablespoon mustard seeds
½ teaspoon sea salt

1. Combine all the ingredients in a stainless steel or enamelled saucepan and bring to a boil. Reduce heat and simmer, uncovered, for 1 hour. Ladle into hot, sterilized jars, wipe the rims, and seal with canning lids. Process in boiling water for 15 minutes. Cool.

2. Refrigerate once opened. Store unopened jars in a cool, dark place.

Carrot and Mustard Seed Relish

Serves 4 to 6

1 pound carrots, peeled and grated
2 tablespoons safflower or vegetable oil
½ teaspoon black mustard seeds
1 or 2 hot green chilies, seeded and sliced (optional)
1 tablespoon chopped fresh coriander
Juice of 1 to 2 lemons, to taste
Sea salt to taste

1. Heat the oil in a large, heavy-bottomed frying pan and add the mustard seeds. Sauté over medium-high heat until they turn gray and stop sputtering. Add the chili pepper, stir a few seconds, and toss with the carrots in a bowl.

2. Season the carrots to taste with sea salt and lemon juice, toss with the coriander, and chill. Serve as a side dish with grain and vegetable dishes or as a salad.

Sweet and Spicy Coriander Sauce

This intriguing sauce could be used as a dip for crudités, or spread on bread, or used as a sauce for vegetables. You could thin it out with more oil, or water from the prunes, for a thinner sauce for grains or pasta. It will keep for several days in the refrigerator.

Makes 1⅓ cups

6 pitted prunes
1 cup fresh coriander leaves, tightly packed
½ cup chopped, fresh parsley
¼ cup fresh lime juice
2 cloves garlic, peeled
½ teaspoon chopped fresh ginger
¼ teaspoon sea salt
¼ teaspoon freshly ground pepper
¼ cup sesame tahini
2 to 4 tablespoons olive or safflower oil

1. Place the prunes in a saucepan and cover with 2 cups water. Bring to a simmer and simmer 15 minutes. Drain and retain the cooking liquid.

2. Combine all the ingredients except the oil and prune water in a blender or food processor fitted with the steel blade and blend together until you have a paste. Without stopping the blender or food processor, blend in the oil and enough of the prune water to give it the consistency you desire. This will depend on whether you wish to use the sauce as a dip, spread, or sauce. The amount of oil or prune water you add will also depend on the consistency of your tahini. If it is very runny, you will need less oil, but if it is thick like peanut butter, you will need more liquid.

3. Store the sauce in a covered jar in the refrigerator.

Mint and Coriander Dip or Chutney

Makes 1¼ cups

¾ cup fresh coriander leaves
½ cup fresh mint leaves
3 tablespoons water
¾ cup plain low-fat yogurt
1 small hot green chili, seeded and minced
1 tablespoon lemon juice
½ teaspoon mild-flavored honey
Sea salt to taste

1. Blend together the coriander and mint with the water in a blender or food processor.
2. Beat the yogurt with a whisk until smooth and stir in the remaining ingredients. Chill.

Ginger Tea

This infusion is very strong, and you can temper it with added water and/or honey.

Serves 4

2-inch piece fresh ginger root, peeled and chopped
3 tablespoons mild-flavored honey (more to taste)
4 cups water
1 stick cinnamon
4 cloves

1. Combine all the ingredients in a saucepan and bring to a boil.
2. Reduce heat, cover, and simmer 30 minutes.
3. Strain, correct sweetening, and serve, or chill and serve. Dilute with water if too strong.

Iced Ginger-Lime Tea

Serves 2

Combine the water, honey, and ginger in a saucepan and bring to a simmer. Simmer 15 minutes and strain. Add the lime or lemon juice. Correct sweetening. Fill glasses with ice cubes and pour in the tea, or chill the ginger-water infusion and combine with the lemon or lime juice just before serving.

2 cups water
1-inch piece fresh ginger root, peeled and chopped
2 tablespoons mild-flavored honey (more to taste)
½ cup lime or lemon juice
Ice cubes

Thandai (Indian Summer Punch)

This is a rather exotic drink that is very popular in India.

Serves 4

1. Place the almonds in a bowl and pour on boiling water to cover. Let sit ½ hour.
2. Grind all the spices together to a fine powder.
3. Combine the almonds, spices, honey, and 1 cup of boiling water in a blender. Blend until thoroughly smooth, and pour into a bowl. Add another ½ cup of water to the blender and turn on to clean the blades and sides. Add to the mixture in the bowl. Strain this through cheesecloth, and chill overnight or for several hours.
4. Combine equal parts of the chilled mixture with milk (ice water may be substituted). Serve very cold.

½ cup blanched almonds
1 tablespoon fennel seeds
Seeds from 4 cardamom pods
3 cloves
3 tablespoons mild-flavored honey
2 cups milk or water

SPICED MINTY YOGURT DRINK

Serves 2

1 cup yogurt or buttermilk
½ cup water
12 mint leaves
½ teaspoon cumin
8 ice cubes
Whole fresh mint leaves for garnish

1. Blend together all the ingredients except the ice cubes and whole mint leaves for the garnish until smooth in a blender.

2. Add the ice cubes and continue to blend another 20 to 30 seconds. Pour into glasses and garnish with the mint leaves. Serve.

SPICED INDIAN TEA

Serves 4 to 6

2 tablespoons dark tea leaves, such as Darjeeling, Assam, or Ceylon
8 white or green cardamom pods
A 2-inch stick cinnamon
4 whole cloves
5 cups water
Honey or milk, to taste

1. Warm the teapot with boiling water, empty, and place in it the tea and spices.

2. Bring the 5 cups of water to a boil and pour into the teapot. Let steep 5 minutes, stir, and serve, adding honey and/or hot milk to taste.

APPLE SMOOTHIE

Serves 2

Blend all the ingredients together in a blender until smooth and frothy. Serve.

1 cup plain low-fat yogurt
1 cup apple juice
2 apples, cored and chopped
1 teaspoon cinnamon
½ teaspoon nutmeg
1 teaspoon vanilla
1 banana, peeled, coarsely chopped
2 teaspoons mild-flavored honey
6 ice cubes

9
DESSERTS

Tofu Cheesecake

Serves 8

For the Crust:
½ cup granola
½ cup wheat germ (or use all granola)
1 teaspoon cinnamon
2 tablespoons melted butter
Additional butter for the pan

For the Filling:
1½ pounds tofu
1 cup plain low-fat yogurt
2 eggs
¾ cup mild-flavored honey
Juice of 2 medium lemons (⅓ cup lemon juice)
Grated rind of 1 lemon
1 tablespoon vanilla
1 teaspoon nutmeg
1 teaspoon cinnamon
2 tablespoons sesame tahini
¼ cup Grand Marnier (optional)
¼ teaspoon sea salt
3 tablespoons whole wheat pastry flour

1. First make the crust. Combine the granola, wheat germ, and cinnamon. Stir in the melted butter. Butter an 8- or 10-inch springform pan or a 10-inch pie pan generously and pour in the granola mixture. Tilt the pan so that some of the mixture adheres to the sides, and layer the rest evenly over the bottom. Refrigerate while you prepare the filling.

2. Preheat the oven to 350°F.

3. Purée all the filling ingredients together in a blender or food processor fitted with the steel blade until completely smooth. Pour into the prepared pan and bake in the preheated oven for 50 to 60 minutes, or until just beginning to brown.

4. Turn off the heat and leave in the oven 30 minutes. Remove from the oven, cool, and chill.

TOFU-BANANA CREAM PIE

Serves 8

1 granola piecrust (see tofu cheesecake, page 180)
1 pound tofu
1½ cups plain low-fat yogurt
⅓ cup mild-flavored honey
2 teaspoons vanilla
1 teaspoon nutmeg
¼ teaspoon sea salt
3 tablespoons whole wheat pastry flour
2 eggs
3 medium or large bananas
Juice of 1 to 2 lemons, to taste
1 additional tablespoon lemon juice
1 cup fresh strawberries, for garnish (optional)

1. Preheat the oven to 350°F. Prepare the granola piecrust as for tofu cheesecake.

2. Slice the bananas and toss in 1 tablespoon lemon juice. Set aside 8 slices for decorating the pie.

3. Liquefy all the remaining filling ingredients, except the bananas you have set aside and the strawberries, in a blender or food processor fitted with the steel blade. Make sure the mixture is completely smooth.

4. Pour the filling into the piecrust and bake 30 minutes in the preheated oven. Turn off the heat and allow the pie to cool in the oven for 30 minutes. Remove from the oven and decorate the top with the reserved banana slices and the optional strawberries. Cover and chill.

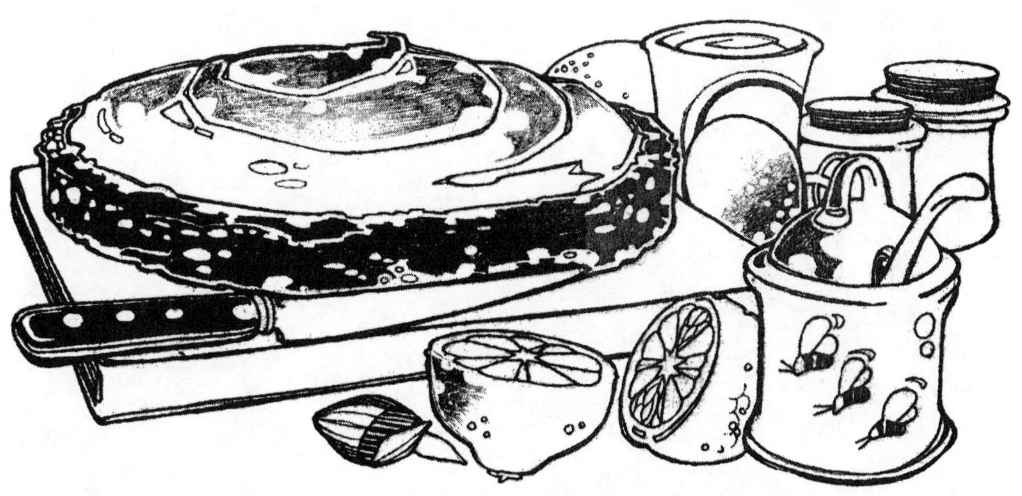

GINGERBREAD

8 servings

3 eggs
½ cup dark molasses
½ cup mild-flavored honey
1 tablespoon ground ginger
1 teaspoon cinnamon
½ teaspoon allspice
½ teaspoon nutmeg
¼ teaspoon sea salt
Grated zest of 1 orange
2 cups whole wheat pastry flour
1 teaspoon baking soda
3 ounces unsalted butter, melted
½ cup plain low-fat yogurt or buttermilk

1. Preheat the oven to 350°F. Butter and lightly flour an 8-inch square baking pan.

2. Beat the eggs until light and frothy. Add the molasses and honey and continue to beat for a minute or two. Beat in the spices, sea salt, and orange zest.

3. Sift together the flours and baking soda. Gradually add 1 cup to the batter, beating slowly. Add the butter and yogurt or buttermilk, then the remaining flour. Mix just until blended.

4. Pour into the prepared pan and bake in the preheated oven about 45 minutes, or until the gingerbread has shrunk from the sides of the pan and a tester inserted in the center comes out clean. Remove from the oven and cool on a rack. Served topped with whipped cream or yogurt.

Baked Apples

Serves 4

4 tart apples
½ cup apple juice
1 teaspoon cinnamon
½ teaspoon freshly grated nutmeg
¼ teaspoon ground cloves
1 teaspoon unsalted butter
2 teaspoons vanilla extract
3 tablespoons raisins
2 tablespoons sunflower seeds or slivered almonds
Plain low-fat yogurt for topping

1. Preheat the oven to 350°F. Lightly butter a baking dish.

2. Cut a cone-shaped cavity into the stem end of each apple and spoon a tablespoon of apple juice into each one. Combine the spices and sprinkle into the cavities. Add ½ teaspoon vanilla extract, then fill each apple with the raisins and sunflower seeds or almonds. Top with ¼ teaspoon butter. Add the remaining apple juice to the pan.

3. Bake in a preheated oven until tender, about 45 minutes, basting from time to time with the apple juice in the pan.

APPLE CRISP

Serves 6

6 tart apples
Juice of 1 lemon
2 tablespoons mild-flavored honey
1 teaspoon cinnamon
½ teaspoon nutmeg
¼ teaspoon cloves
2 tablespoons sunflower seeds
1 tablespoon cornstarch dissolved in 2 tablespoons water
2 teaspoons vanilla

For the Topping:
1½ cups rolled oats
½ cup whole wheat flour
¼ teaspoon sea salt
2 teaspoons cinnamon
1 teaspoon allspice
6 tablespoons unsalted butter or safflower oil
⅓ cup mild-flavored honey

1. Preheat the oven to 375°F. Oil or butter a 2-quart baking dish.

2. Combine the apples, lemon juice, honey, cinnamon, nutmeg, cloves, sunflower seeds, cornstarch dissolved in the water, and vanilla. Spread evenly in the prepared baking dish.

3. Using a food processor, or in a bowl with a wooden spoon, mix together the ingredients for the topping and combine well. Spread evenly over the apple mixture.

4. Bake in the preheated oven for 30 to 45 minutes, or until the top is brown and crisp. Serve warm, topped with plain low-fat yogurt.

Apple Sauce

Serves 4 to 6

1. Combine all the ingredients in a saucepan and simmer together over low heat for 45 minutes to an hour, stirring from time to time with a wooden spoon, until the mixture is thoroughly softened.
2. Mash to a purée with the back of a spoon. Eat warm or chilled, plain, with yogurt, or as a spread on toast. This also makes a nice snack.

6 tart apples, cored and chopped
½ cup water or apple juice
2 tablespoons mild-flavored honey
1 teaspoon cinnamon
½ teaspoon nutmeg
¼ teaspoon ground cloves
¼ teaspoon allspice
Juice of 1 lemon

Dried Fruit Compote with Yogurt

Serves 4 to 6

1. Place all the ingredients except the nutmeg and yogurt or cream in a large saucepan and bring to a boil. Reduce heat, cover, and simmer 30 minutes.
2. Sprinkle with freshly grated nutmeg and serve topped with plain low-fat yogurt or whipped cream.

1 cup dried apricots
1 cup prunes
½ cup raisins
½ cup chopped dried pears or peaches
1 stick cinnamon
4 cloves
2 cups water
2 cups red wine
4 tablespoons mild-flavored honey
Freshly grated nutmeg to taste
1 cup plain low-fat yogurt or whipped cream

BAKED PEARS

Serves 4 to 6

4 to 6 pears, peeled, cored, and quartered
½ cup apple juice
¼ teaspoon cinnamon
¼ teaspoon freshly grated nutmeg
Plain low-fat yogurt for topping (optional)

1. Preheat the oven to 350°F.

2. Place the peeled, cored, and quartered pears in a baking dish and pour in the apple juice. Sprinkle with cinnamon and nutmeg and cover the dish with foil or a lid.

3. Bake in the preheated oven for 30 minutes, or until the pears are soft but not mushy, and are aromatic. Serve hot or cool, with a spoonful or two of the apple juice. Top, if you wish, with plain low-fat yogurt.

GRAPEFRUIT AND FIGS WITH GINGER AND LIME

Serves 4 to 6

8 fresh figs, quartered or cut in half
3 pink grapefruit, peeled, white pith removed, and sectioned
⅓ cup lime juice
4 tablespoons mild-flavored honey
2 teaspoons minced fresh ginger
¼ teaspoon cinnamon

1. Toss together the figs and grapefruit.

2. Mix together the lime juice, honey, ginger, and cinnamon. Toss with the fruit and serve, or chill and serve.

Peaches in Red Wine

Serves 4 to 6

4 to 6 ripe peaches, peeled, pitted, and sliced
3 cups red wine
4 tablespoons mild-flavored honey
1 teaspoon cinnamon

1. Blanch the peaches, run under cold water, and gently remove the skins.

2. Combine the wine, honey, and cinnamon in a bowl. Slice the peaches and add to this mixture. Cover and chill. Serve cold.

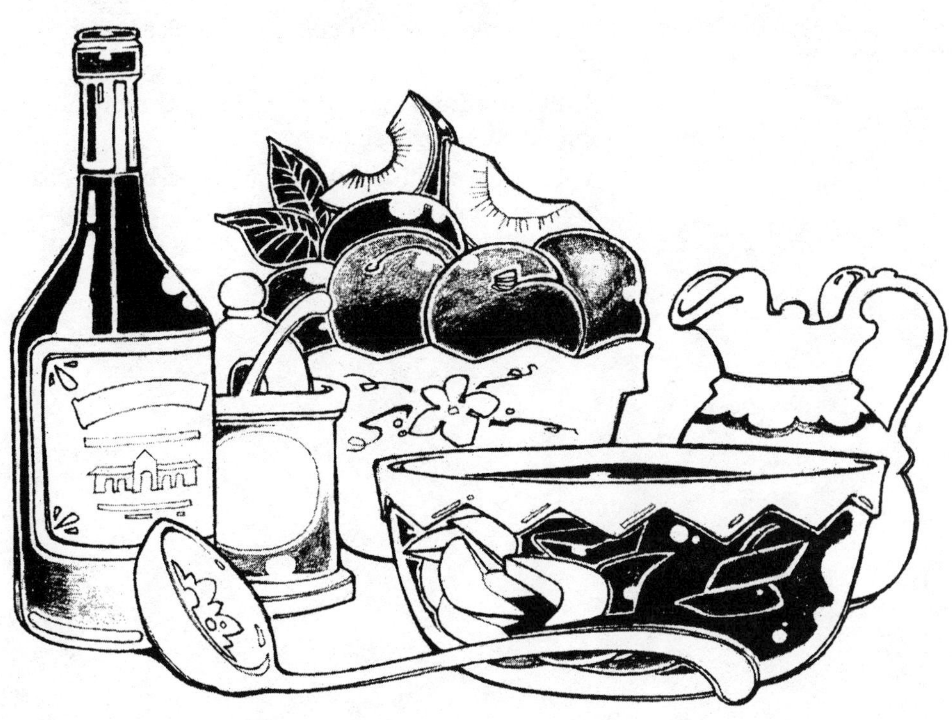

Indian Pudding

This is adapted from my cookbook *The Vegetarian Feast.*

Serves 6 to 8

1 quart milk, scalded
6 tablespoons stone-ground yellow cornmeal
⅓ cup molasses
3 tablespoons mild-flavored honey
4 eggs, beaten
½ teaspoon sea salt
1 teaspoon ground ginger
½ teaspoon freshly grated nutmeg
3 tablespoons butter
½ cup raisins

1. Preheat the oven to 325°F. Butter a 2-quart casserole or soufflé dish.

2. Bring the milk to the boiling point in a 2- or 3-quart saucepan. Pour in the cornmeal in a slow stream, stirring all the while with a wooden spoon as if you were making polenta. Bring to a gentle boil and cook over low heat, stirring, for about 15 minutes, or until the mixture is thick and creamy. Add the molasses and honey and cook another 5 minutes.

3. Remove from the heat and stir in the remaining ingredients. Mix well.

4. Pour the pudding into the prepared baking dish and bake for 1 to 1½ hours in the preheated oven, or until a knife comes out clean and the top is just beginning to brown.

Cherry Clafouti

Serves 6

1½ pounds pitted cherries
1¼ cups milk
4 tablespoons mild-flavored honey
3 eggs
1 tablespoon vanilla
¼ teaspoon nutmeg
Pinch of sea salt
⅓ cup unbleached white flour
⅓ cup whole wheat pastry flour
2 tablespoons kirsch
Plain low-fat yogurt or cream for topping

1. Pit the cherries and retain any liquid.

2. Place the milk, the liquid from the cherries, honey, eggs, vanilla, nutmeg, and salt in a blender and turn it on. Add the flours while the blender is running. Blend for 1 minute. If mixing by hand, blend together the eggs and flour with a wooden spoon and whisk or beat in the liquids. Strain through a fine strainer and stir in the kirsch. Let the batter rest for 30 minutes.

3. Preheat the oven to 350°F. Butter a 2-quart flameproof baking dish and pour in a ¼-inch layer of batter. Place over moderate heat for 1 to 2 minutes, or just until a film has set on the bottom. Now spread the cherries in an even layer and pour on the remaining batter.

4. Place in the preheated oven and bake 45 minutes, or until puffed and brown and a knife plunged into the center comes out clean. Serve hot or warm, with a little cream or yogurt to moisten.

Mangoes, Kiwi, and Pineapple in Syrup

Serves 6 to 8

For the Syrup:
1 quart water
½ cup mild-flavored honey
1 clove
½ teaspoon Chinese Five Spice powder
Grated zest of 2 limes
Grated zest of 1 lemon
1½ vanilla beans, split in half
1 teaspoon minced fresh ginger
3 coriander seeds
1 sprig mint

For the Fruit:
2 large mangoes, peeled, seeded, and diced
½ fresh, ripe pineapple, peeled, cored, and diced
8 kiwis, peeled and sliced
1 tablespoon chopped fresh mint

1. First make the syrup. Combine all the ingredients in a large saucepan and bring to a boil. Remove from the heat and allow to cool. Cover and chill for several hours.

2. Place the fruit in a serving bowl. Strain in the syrup. Toss gently and cover. Refrigerate for at least 2 hours.

3. Just before serving toss with the mint.

GINGERSNAPS

Makes 4 to 5 dozen

6 ounces butter
6 tablespoons mild-flavored honey
½ cup molasses
1 egg
2½ cups whole wheat pastry flour
¼ teaspoon sea salt
1 teaspoon ground cinnamon
¼ teaspoon freshly ground pepper
1 tablespoon ground ginger

1. Preheat the oven to 350°F. Butter baking sheets.

2. Cream together the butter, honey, and molasses, and beat in the egg. Sift together the whole wheat pastry flour, sea salt, cinnamon, pepper, and ground ginger. Add to the liquid ingredients and mix well.

3. Drop by scant tablespoons onto the baking sheets, about 2 inches apart. Take a glass or jar and dip the bottom into cool water, then press out the cookies very thin. Keep wetting the glass to avoid sticking.

4. Bake for 10 to 12 minutes; cool on racks.

BIBLIOGRAPHY AND SUGGESTED READING

Cost, Bruce, *Ginger, East to West,* Aris Books, Berkeley, Los Angeles, 1984.

David, Elizabeth, *Spices, Salt and Aromatics in the English Kitchen,* Penguin Books, London and New York, 1970.

David, Elizabeth, *English Bread and Yeast Cookery,* The Viking Press, London and New York, 1980.

Jaffrey, Madhur, *An Invitation to Indian Cooking,* Jonathan Cape, London, 1976.

Jaffrey, Madhur, *World of the East Vegetarian Cooking,* Alfred A. Knopf & Co., New York, 1981.

Kennedy, Diane, *The Cuisines of Mexico,* Harper & Row, Publishers, New York, 1972.

Rosengarten, Frederick Jr., *The Book of Spices,* Jove Publications, Inc., New York, 1973.

Sahni, Julie, *Classic Indian Cooking,* William Morrow & Co., Inc., New York, 1980.

Sax, Richard, *Cooking Great Meals Every Day,* Random House, New York, 1982.

Sax, Richard, *Old Fashioned Desserts,* Irena Chalmers Cookbooks, Inc., New York, 1984.

Scott, David, *Middle Eastern Vegetarian Cookery,* Rider & Co., Ltd, London, 1981.

Shulman, Martha Rose, *Herb and Honey Cookery,* Thorsons Publishers Ltd, Wellingborough and New York, 1984.

Stobart, Tom, *Herbs, Spices and Flavorings,* Penguin Books, London, 1977.

Tropp, Barbara, 'All About Peppercorns,' in *Food and Wine,* May, 1985.

INDEX